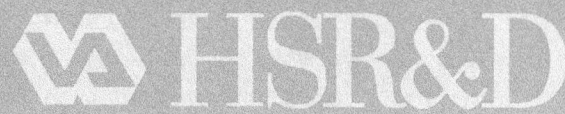

I0470830

Safe and Effective Anticoagulation in the Outpatient Setting: A Systematic Review of the Evidence

February 2011

Prepared for:
Department of Veterans Affairs
Veterans Health Administration
Health Services Research & Development Service
Washington, DC 20420

Prepared by:
VA Evidence-based Synthesis Program (ESP) Center
Center for Chronic Disease Outcomes Research
Minneapolis VA Medical Center
Minneapolis, MN
Timothy J. Wilt, MD, MPH, Director

Investigators:
Principal Investigators:
Hanna E. Bloomfield, MD, MPH
Brent C. Taylor, PhD, MPH

Co-Investigators:
Ange Krause, MD
Preetham Reddy, MD

Research Associates:
Nancy Greer, PhD
Roderick MacDonald, MS
Indulis Rutks, BA

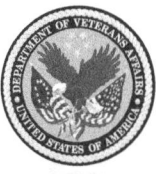

PREFACE

Health Services Research & Development Service's (HSR&D's) Evidence-based Synthesis Program (ESP) was established to provide timely and accurate syntheses of targeted healthcare topics of particular importance to Veterans Affairs (VA) managers and policymakers, as they work to improve the health and healthcare of Veterans. The ESP disseminates these reports throughout VA.

HSR&D provides funding for four ESP Centers and each Center has an active VA affiliation. The ESP Centers generate evidence syntheses on important clinical practice topics, and these reports help:

- develop clinical policies informed by evidence,
- guide the implementation of effective services to improve patient outcomes and to support VA clinical practice guidelines and performance measures, and
- set the direction for future research to address gaps in clinical knowledge.

In 2009, the ESP Coordinating Center was created to expand the capacity of HSR&D Central Office and the four ESP sites by developing and maintaining program processes. In addition, the Center established a Steering Committee comprised of HSR&D field-based investigators, VA Patient Care Services, Office of Quality and Performance, and Veterans Integrated Service Networks (VISN) Clinical Management Officers. The Steering Committee provides program oversight, guides strategic planning, coordinates dissemination activities, and develops collaborations with VA leadership to identify new ESP topics of importance to Veterans and the VA healthcare system.

Comments on this evidence report are welcome and can be sent to Nicole Floyd, ESP Coordinating Center Program Manager, at nicole.floyd@va.gov.

Recommended citation: Bloomfield HE, Taylor BC, Krause A, Reddy P, Greer N, MacDonald R, Rutks, I, Wilt, T. Safe and Effective Anticoagulation in the Outpatient Setting: A Systematic Review of the Evidence. VA-ESP Project #09-009; 2011

This report is based on research conducted by the Evidence-based Synthesis Program (ESP) Center located at the Minneapolis VA Medical Center, Minneapolis, MN funded by the Department of Veterans Affairs, Veterans Health Administration, Office of Research and Development, Health Services Research and Development. The findings and conclusions in this document are those of the author(s) who are responsible for its contents; the findings and conclusions do not necessarily represent the views of the Department of Veterans Affairs or the United States government. Therefore, no statement in this article should be construed as an official position of the Department of Veterans Affairs. No investigators have any affiliations or financial involvement (e.g., employment, consultancies, honoraria, stock ownership or options, expert testimony, grants or patents received or pending, or royalties) that conflict with material presented in the report.

TABLE OF CONTENTS

FIGURES

EXECUTIVE SUMMARY

BACKGROUND

Long term anticoagulation with Vitamin K antagonists (e.g., warfarin) has been shown to reduce major thromboembolic complications in patients with many common chronic conditions, including atrial fibrillation, history of deep vein thrombosis and pulmonary embolism, and mechanical heart valves. However, Vitamin K antagonists have a very narrow therapeutic window requiring frequent laboratory monitoring to ensure that patients are neither excessively anti-coagulated, which increases the risk for bleeding, or under anti-coagulated, which increases the risk for thromboembolism. Laboratory monitoring consists of measuring the blood's tendency to clot with a test known as the International Normalized Ratio (INR), usually performed every 4-6 weeks. Dosage adjustments are then based on these results.

Since management of long term oral anticoagulation requires frequent testing and dose adjustment, anticoagulation clinics (ACC) have been developed to streamline and standardize this care. Typically run by specially trained nurses or pharmacists, these clinics provide intense patient education and timely follow-up of INR results, use algorithms for dose adjustments, and are easily accessible to patients between visits. More recently, portable devices have become available that are able to accurately measure the INR with a drop of capillary blood. This means that patients can now test themselves at home and either call in the result to their provider who suggests dosage adjustments (known as patient self testing, PST) or adjust their dose of medication themselves (known as patient self management, PSM).

It should be noted that new anticoagulants which may offer the same clinical efficacy and safety profile as warfarin with considerable less monitoring are currently being evaluated for the US market. Final FDA approval of these products may significantly alter the standard for anticoagulation therapy and subsequent monitoring.

OBJECTIVES

The primary objectives of this systematic review were to: 1. Determine whether specialized anticoagulation clinics (ACC) are more effective and safer than care in non-specialized clinics (e.g., primary care clinics, physician offices) for management of long- term anticoagulation in adults; 2. Determine whether patient self testing (PST), either alone or in combination with patient self management (PSM), is more effective and safer than standard care; and 3. Identify the risk factors for serious bleeding in patients on chronic anticoagulant therapy.

METHODS

We searched OVID MEDLINE for relevant articles published in peer-reviewed journals from 1997 to March, 2010 (October, 2010 for Key Question 2) that involved an outpatient, adult population receiving chronic anti-coagulation therapy. We excluded non-English publications and case series, case reports, qualitative reports, narrative reviews, and editorials or letters. Full-text versions of potentially relevant articles were obtained for further review and trained researchers extracted data from articles that met inclusion criteria. The quality of the individual randomized studies was assessed by standard criteria. Analyses of pooled data using a DerSimonian and Laird random-effects model were conducted for outcomes in Key Question 1. Due to low event rates for several clinical outcomes, Peto odds ratios (a fixed-effects model) were calculated for outcomes in Key Question 2.

RESULTS

Key Question 1

For management of long-term outpatient anticoagulation in adults, are specialized anticoagulation clinics (ACC) more effective and safer than care in non-specialized clinics (e.g., primary care clinics, physician offices)?

Overview of Included Studies

We identified a total of 11 articles reporting on 3 randomized clinical trials (RCTs) and 8 cohort studies that met all inclusion criteria. A total of 722 subjects were enrolled in the 3 RCTs which were conducted in the US, China, and Canada. The mean age of subjects enrolled in the RCTs was 68 years (range of study means 59 to 76). A total of 12,768 subjects were included in the 8 observational studies. The mean age of subjects enrolled in the cohort studies was 69 years (range of study means, 57 to 74). Five of the 8 cohort studies were conducted in the US and 3 in other countries. Three studies were prospective and 5 were retrospective cohort studies.

Clinical outcomes in the RCTs

Rates of all-cause mortality, major thromboembolic events, and major bleeding did not differ significantly between the two treatment arms in any of the 3 RCTs. In the pooled analysis, there were 5 deaths in the ACC group and 6 in the Usual Care (UC) group, all from a single study (RR: 0.81, 95%CI: 0.25 to 2.58); 6 major bleeding events in the ACC patients and 8 in UC patients (RR: 1.05, 95%CI: 0.36 to 3.12); 11 major thromboembolic events in the ACC and 14 in the UC patients (RR: 1.29, 95%CI: 0.59 to 2.81).

The pooled weighted mean of percent time within therapeutic range (%TTR) for patients randomized to ACC was 59.9% (range of means 56-64%), only slightly higher than the 56.3% (range of means 52 to 59%) for the patients randomized to UC, for a weighted mean difference of 3.6% (range of mean differences, 3.3 to 5%).

Clinical Outcomes in the Cohort Studies

In the one study reporting all-cause mortality there was no significant difference between ACC and UC. In the 4 studies reporting major thromboembolic events, 1 reported a significantly higher incidence in UC, 1 a significantly higher incidence in ACC, and in 2 studies, p values were not reported. The incidence of major bleeding events was reported in 5 studies and was significantly higher in UC in 1, and not significantly different between groups in 1. Significance testing was not included for the 3 other studies that reported this outcome. We were unable to pool major clinical outcomes because outcomes were reported as number of events in only 2 of the 8 studies; the other studies reported events per patient- or treatment-year.

The pooled weighted mean of %TTR for the 4 studies reporting this metric, was 63.5% for the intervention groups and 53.5% for the control groups, for a weighted mean difference of 10%

(range of mean differences, 4.3 to 26%).

Conclusion and Recommendation

Evidence for the safety and efficacy of ACC is limited but overall suggests that care provided within ACC may lead to better quality anticoagulation control as measured by time in therapeutic range. There is insufficient evidence to conclude that ACC care leads to fewer deaths, thromboembolic events, or major bleeding events than care provided in usual care settings such as primary care clinics. Results from two studies suggest that patients like the convenience and enhanced service provided by these clinics. There is insufficient evidence for the VA to actively promote the implementation of ACCs.

Key Question 2
Is Patient Self Testing (PST), either alone or in combination with Patient Self Management (PSM), more effective and safer than standard care delivered in either ACCs or non-specialized clinics?

Overview of Included Studies

We identified a total of 27 references reporting on 22 distinct randomized clinical trials. Two studies were conducted in the US, 1 in Canada, and 19 in Europe. Duration of follow-up was less than 12 months in 13 studies and 12 or more months in 9. A total of 8413 subjects were included in the 22 trials, with individual trial sample sizes ranging from 50 to 2922. Five trials met all 4 quality indicators (allocation concealment, blinding, intention to treat analysis, and dropouts reported).

Subjects

The mean age of the subjects was 65 (range of study means 42 to 75 years). The percentage of patients screened who met preliminary eligibility criteria, successfully completed the training, and agreed to enter the study ranged from 10-69%. Among patients who were randomized, the percentage who continued with the intervention throughout the study period ranged from 64-98%.

Interventions

Evaluated interventions included PST only (i.e., dose adjustment made by the clinic) and PST/PSM (i.e., testing and dose adjustment made by patient). The patient self testing/self management intervention usually included 2-4 small group training sessions over several weeks. Training sessions typically included general information on anticoagulation, possible interactions with foods/medicines, how to use the INR testing machine, how to adjust the dose, how often to check INR, and when to call for help. The control group received anticoagulation management in an ACC in 11 of the trials, in a primary care or other physician office in 7 trials, and in multiple settings in 3 trials. The other trial compared PST to PSM without another control group.

Clinical Outcomes

There were 298 deaths in subjects randomized to PST/PSM intervention compared to 369 deaths in the control subjects (Peto OR: 0.74, 95%CI: 0.63 to 0.87, P=0.000), I^2=51%) The intervention group had 283 major bleeding events compared with 300 in the control group (Peto OR: 0.89, 95%CI: 0.75 to 1.05, P =0.169, I^2=2%, There were 99 major thromboembolic events in the intervention group compared with 149 in the control group (Peto OR 0.58, 95%CI: 0.45 to 0.75, P<0.000, I^2=27%).

The pooled weighted mean of time within therapeutic range for patients randomized to PST/PSM interventions was 66.1% (range of means 56-76.5%), which was not significantly different than the 61.9% (range of means 32 to 77%) for the patients randomized to usual care.

The Home INR Study (THINRS)

This trial is of particular interest since it was conducted in the Department of Veterans Affairs (VA) and is the largest trial to date comparing patient self-testing with usual care. The trial randomized 2,922 patients at 28 VA Medical Centers to high quality anticoagulation clinic management or patient self testing. The primary endpoint was time to first event: stroke, major bleed, or death. The time to event curves did not differ significantly between intervention groups for either the primary endpoint or any of its three individual components. Time in target range and patient satisfaction were significantly higher in the PST group.

Conclusion and Recommendation

This review indicates that compared to usual clinic care, patient self testing with or without self management is associated with significantly fewer deaths and thromboembolic events without any increase in bleeding complications, for a select group of motivated patients requiring long term anticoagulation with Vitamin K antagonists. It should be noted, however, that while the strength of evidence was moderate for the thromboembolism and bleeding, it was low for mortality. Whether this care model is cost-effective and can be implemented successfully in typical US health care settings requires further study.

Key Question 3
What are the risk factors for serious bleeding in patients on chronic anticoagulant therapy?

Overview of Included Studies

We identified a total of 35 articles representing 35 unique studies that provided evidence regarding the impact of various risk factors for predicting serious bleeding events. Each article provided a different set of reported risk factors, in a diverse range of patient populations, using different lengths of follow-up. These differences make statistical pooling of results unreliable, so the evidence is summarized in a narrative format.

Subject Characteristics

A total of 453,918 subjects were included in these studies. Studies ranged in size from a case control study with 26 cases to a large administrative database study of Medicare records that included 353,489 patients. Since any averages of patient characteristics across studies will be mostly driven by the few large administrative studies, the value of overall patient characteristics is somewhat limited. Most studies included primarily elderly populations with an average age of approximately 70 years.

Predictors of Serious Bleeding

Many factors have been shown to predict an increased risk of serious bleeding; however, there is no standard set of variables that is commonly reported. Factors that seemed most consistently associated with increased serious bleeding included: very old age, the first months following warfarin initiation, other medication use (particularly aspirin use), comorbid conditions (such as history of gastrointestinal bleeding events or diabetes), patients whose primary indication for taking warfarin was due to valve conditions, variability in INR values, and genetic factors (ex. variation in the CYP2C gene). There have also been a number of studies of indices that pool together several of the before mentioned risk factors. These studies have shown that patients can, to some extent, be categorized into low, intermediate and higher risk for serious bleeding events based on these indices. Those identified as low risk typically have a several-fold lower risk of bleeding events compared to those identified as high risk. The amount of separation depended, in part, on the population. For example, a population where most of the patients are generally at a low risk of major bleeding will tend to show little separation because there is not much of a range in risk.

Conclusion and Recommendation

Several factors have been shown to predict an increased risk of bleeding and when pooled together a subset of these risk factors has been shown to stratify groups of patients into lower and higher risk groups. Either alone or in combination, these risk factors can likely be used to help clinicians and patients have a dialog about the risks of warfarin therapy. Currently, there is not adequate evidence to suggest that any of the bleeding risk indices are meaningfully superior to the other indices. Future studies might better define the utility of these risk indices by randomizing patients to different bleed risk management strategies that incorporate different combinations of risk factors or bleed risk indices to assess the potential benefits and harms of different anti-coagulation strategies.

EVIDENCE REPORT

INTRODUCTION

BACKGROUND AND TOPIC DEVELOPMENT

Long term anticoagulation with Vitamin K antagonists (e.g. warfarin) has been shown to reduce major thromboembolic complications in patients with many common chronic conditions, including atrial fibrillation, history of deep vein thrombosis and pulmonary embolism, and mechanical heart valves. However, Vitamin K antagonists have a very narrow therapeutic window requiring frequent laboratory monitoring to ensure that patients are neither excessively anti-coagulated, which increases the risk for bleeding, or under anti-coagulated, which increases the risk for thromboembolism. Laboratory monitoring consists of measuring the blood's tendency to clot with a test known as the International Normalized Ratio (INR), usually performed every 4-6 weeks. Dosage adjustments are then based on these results.

Since management of long term oral anticoagulation requires frequent testing and dose adjustment, anticoagulation clinics (ACC) have been developed to streamline and standardize this care.[1] Typically run by specially trained nurses or pharmacists, these clinics provide intense patient education, provide timely follow-up of INR results, use algorithms for dose adjustments, and are easily accessible to patients between visits. More recently, portable devices have become available that are able to accurately measure the INR with a drop of capillary blood. This means that patients can now test themselves at home and either call in the result to their provider who suggests dosage adjustments (known as patient self testing, PST) or adjust their dose of medication themselves (known as patient self management, PSM).[2]

As a leader in safety and quality, the Department of Veterans Affairs (VA) is interested in assuring that veterans on long-term anticoagulation receive state-of-the-art care that maximizes efficacy and minimizes complications. Towards that end, this review was commissioned by the VA's Evidence-based Synthesis Program, in conjunction with the Office of Quality and Performance. Rowena Dolor, MD, MHS; Adam Rose, MD, MSc; and Keith Trettin, RPh, MBA agreed to serve on the Technical Expert Panel (TEP) for the project. We conferred with the TEP members and other experts inside and outside the VA to select the parameters of the review, including patient characteristics, interventions, and outcomes (Figure 1, Analytic Framework).

The final key questions are:

1. For management of long-term outpatient anticoagulation in adults, are specialized anticoagulation clinics (ACC) more effective and safer than care in non-specialized clinics (e.g., primary care clinics, physician offices)?

1a. Which components of a specialized anticoagulation clinic are associated with effectiveness/safety?

2. Is Patient Self Testing (PST), either alone or in combination with Patient Self Management (PSM), more effective and safer than standard care delivered in either ACCs or non-specialized clinics?

3. What are the risk factors for serious bleeding in patients on chronic anticoagulant therapy?

Safe and Effective Anticoagulation in the Outpatient Setting

Figure 1 Analytic Framework

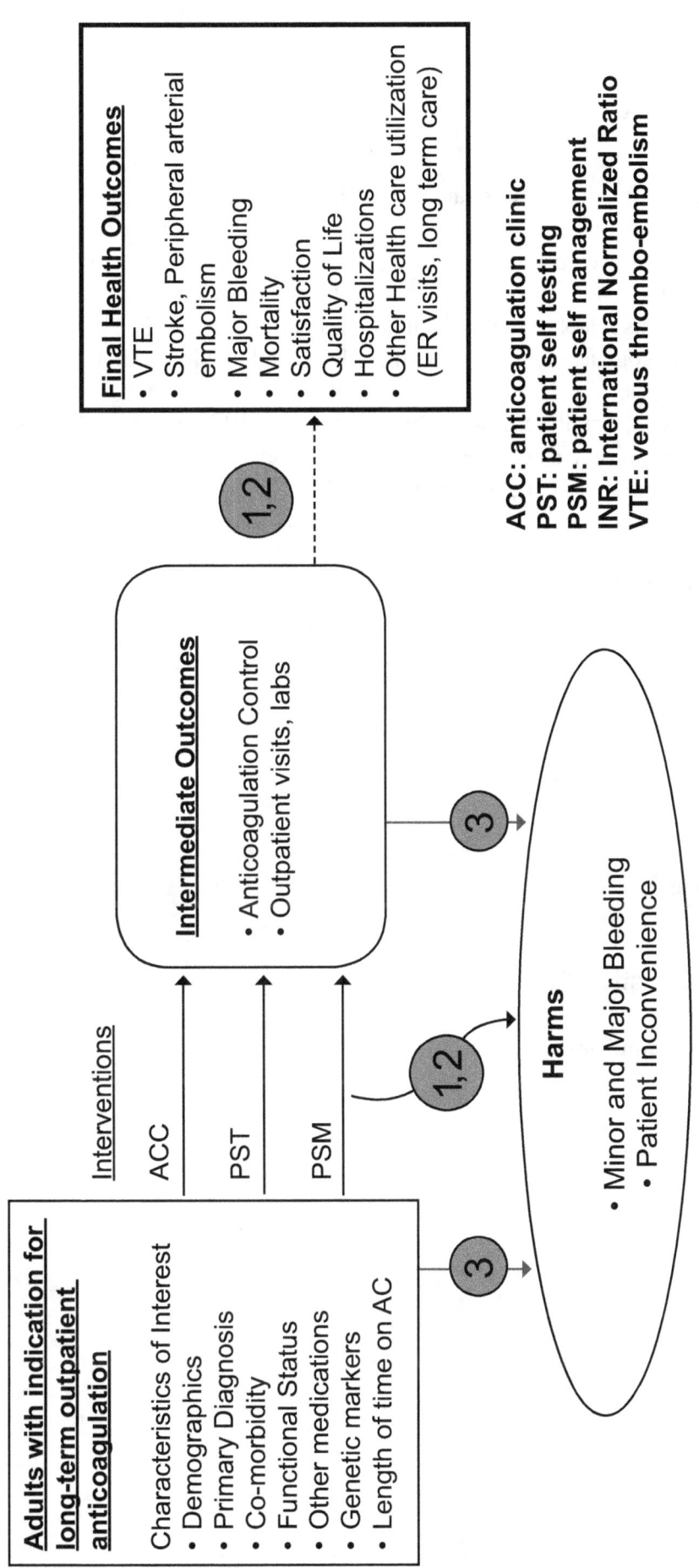

ACC: anticoagulation clinic
PST: patient self testing
PSM: patient self management
INR: International Normalized Ratio
VTE: venous thrombo-embolism

KQ1: For mangement of long term outpatient aniticoagulation in adults, are specialized anticoagulation clinics, (ACC) more effective and safer than care in non-specialized clinics (e.g., primary care clinics, physician offices)?

KQ1a: Which components of a specialized anticoagulation clinic are associated with effectiveness/safety?

KQ2: Are patient self testing (PST) and self management (PSM) effective, safe and cost-effective?

KQ3: What are the risk factors for serious bleeding in patients on chronic anticoagulant therapy?

METHODS

SEARCH STRATEGY

We searched Ovid MEDLINE using the search strategies outlined below. For Key Question 1 we searched the <1950 to 2010> database, downloaded the results and then excluded pre-1996 references. For Key Question 2, we searched the <1950 to 2010> database, limited the results to references from 2005-2010 in the search string and then downloaded the results for further inclusion/exclusion determination. This search was limited to articles published after 2004 because of the availability of a 2007 technology assessment report directly related to this question.[2] For Key Question 3, we searched the <1996 to 2010> database and then downloaded the results for further inclusion/exclusion determination. For all three Key Questions, the initial literature search was completed in 2009. All searches were updated in March 2010 using identical search strategies. The literature search for Key Question 2 was updated again in October 2010. We also searched the Cochrane Library and identified additional citations from reference lists of relevant articles.

Search Strategy – Key Question #1:

1 warfarin.mp. or exp Warfarin/
2 coumadin.mp.
3 coumarin.mp. or exp Coumarins/
4 exp anticoagulants/ or anticoagul*.mp.
5 or/1-4
6 Ambulatory Care Facilities/
7 Outpatient Clinics, Hospital/
8 6 or 7
9 5 and 8
10 (anticoagul* adj clinic*).mp.
11 9 or 10

Search Strategy – Key Question #2:

1 exp anticoagulants/
2 (warfarin or coumadin or coumarin).mp.
3 (oral adj anticoagul$).mp.
4 or/1-3
5 self administration/
6 drug administration schedule/
7 international normalized ratio/
8 near patient test$.mp.
9 point of care systems/
10 self test$.mp.
11 self manage$.mp.
12 drug monitoring/
13 primary health care/
14 (primary care or general practice or general practitioner$).mp.
15 or/5-14
16 4 and 15
17 limit 16 to yr="2005 -Current"

Search Strategy – Key Question #3:

1 (warfarin or coumadin or coumarin).mp.
2 exp HEMORRHAGE/ or hemorrhag*.mp.
3 exp CEREBROVASCULAR ACCIDENT/
4 exp CEREBROVASCULAR TRAUMA/
5 bleed$.mp.
6 stroke.mp.
7 or/2-6
8 1 and 7
9 risk factor*.mp. or exp Risk Factors/
10 predict*.mp. or exp Risk/
11 9 or 10
12 8 and 11
13 cohort stud*.mp. or exp Cohort Studies/
14 prospective stud*.mp. or exp Prospective Studies/
15 random*.mp. or exp Randomized Controlled Trial/
16 or/13-15
17 12 and 16

Trained researchers reviewed the titles and abstracts identified by the literature search to identify articles published in the English language, in peer-reviewed journals, and related to one of the key questions. For KQ1 and KQ2, we included articles that involved an outpatient, adult population receiving chronic (defined as more than 3 months) anti-coagulation therapy. For KQ3, we further limited the inclusion criteria to studies that involved warfarin therapy, reported results by risk factor status, and had a study population of at least 25 cases of serious bleeding. For all questions, we excluded case series, case reports, qualitative reports, narrative reviews, and editorials or letters. Full-text versions of potentially relevant articles were obtained for further review (see Figures 2, 3, and 4) and trained researchers extracted data from articles that met inclusion criteria.

Figure 2. Literature Flow Diagram for Key Question 1

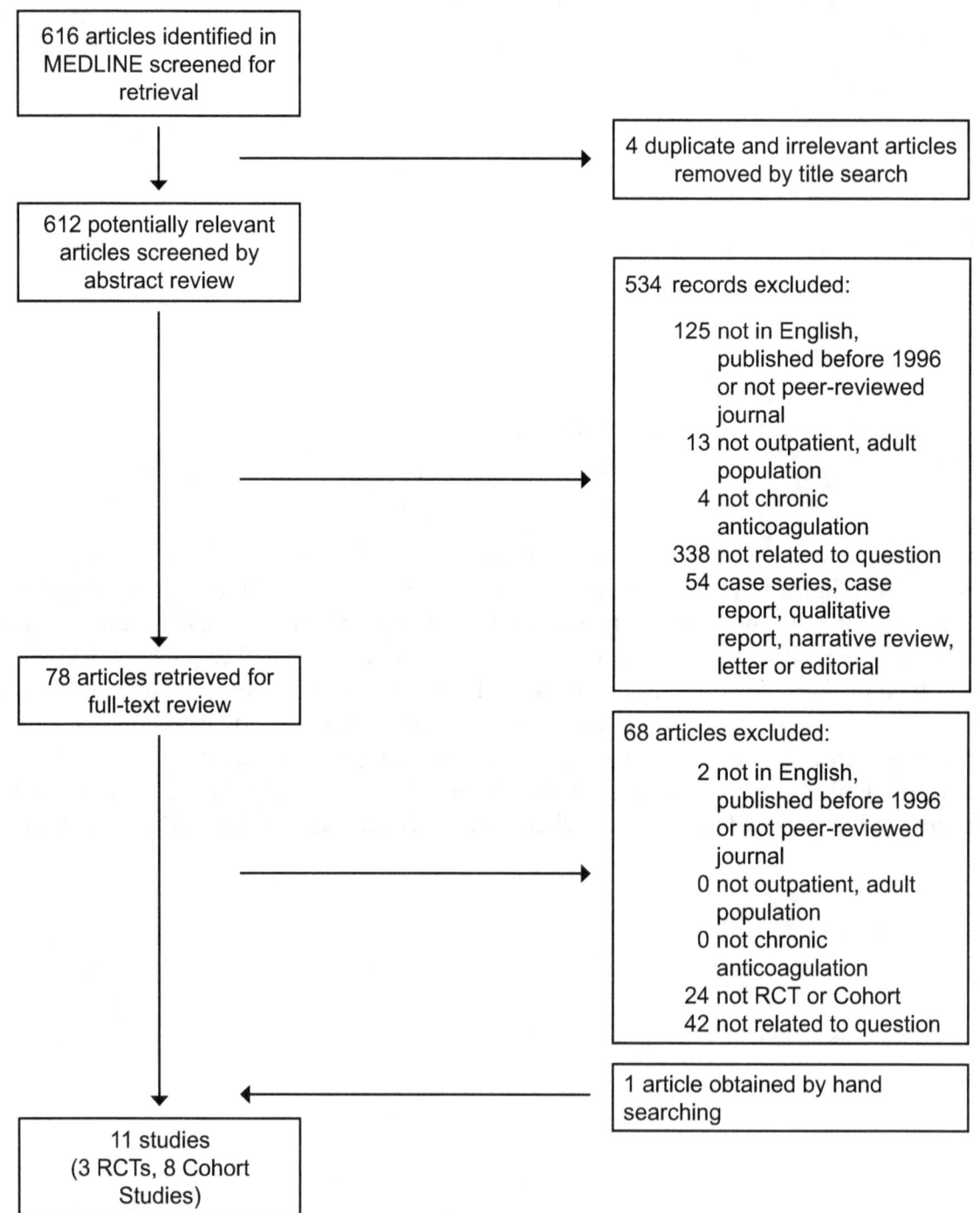

Figure 3. Literature Flow Diagram for Key Question 2

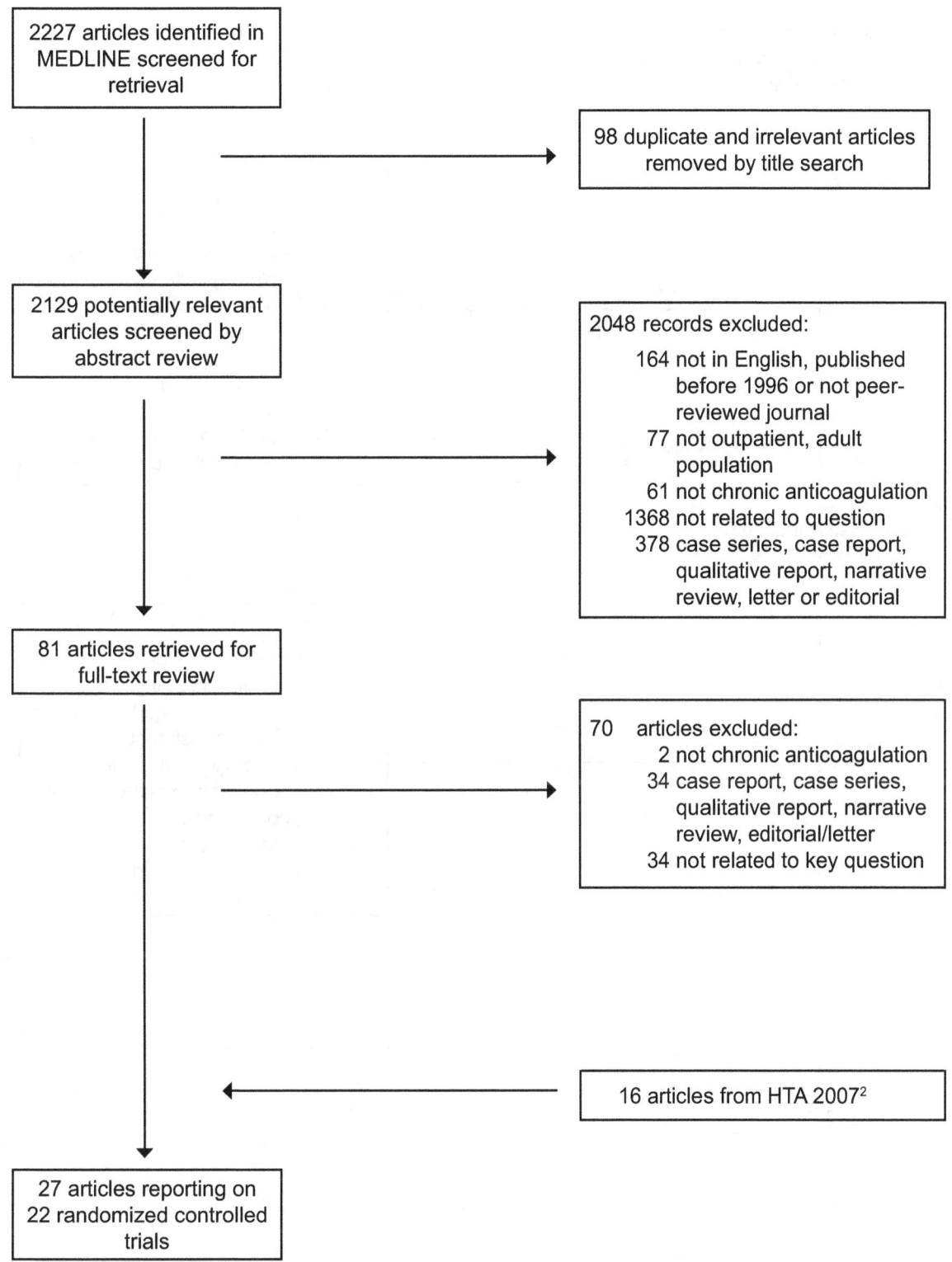

2227 articles identified in MEDLINE screened for retrieval

98 duplicate and irrelevant articles removed by title search

2129 potentially relevant articles screened by abstract review

2048 records excluded:

164 not in English, published before 1996 or not peer-reviewed journal
77 not outpatient, adult population
61 not chronic anticoagulation
1368 not related to question
378 case series, case report, qualitative report, narrative review, letter or editorial

81 articles retrieved for full-text review

70 articles excluded:

2 not chronic anticoagulation
34 case report, case series, qualitative report, narrative review, editorial/letter
34 not related to key question

16 articles from HTA 2007[2]

27 articles reporting on 22 randomized controlled trials

Figure 4. Literature Flow Diagram for Key Question 3

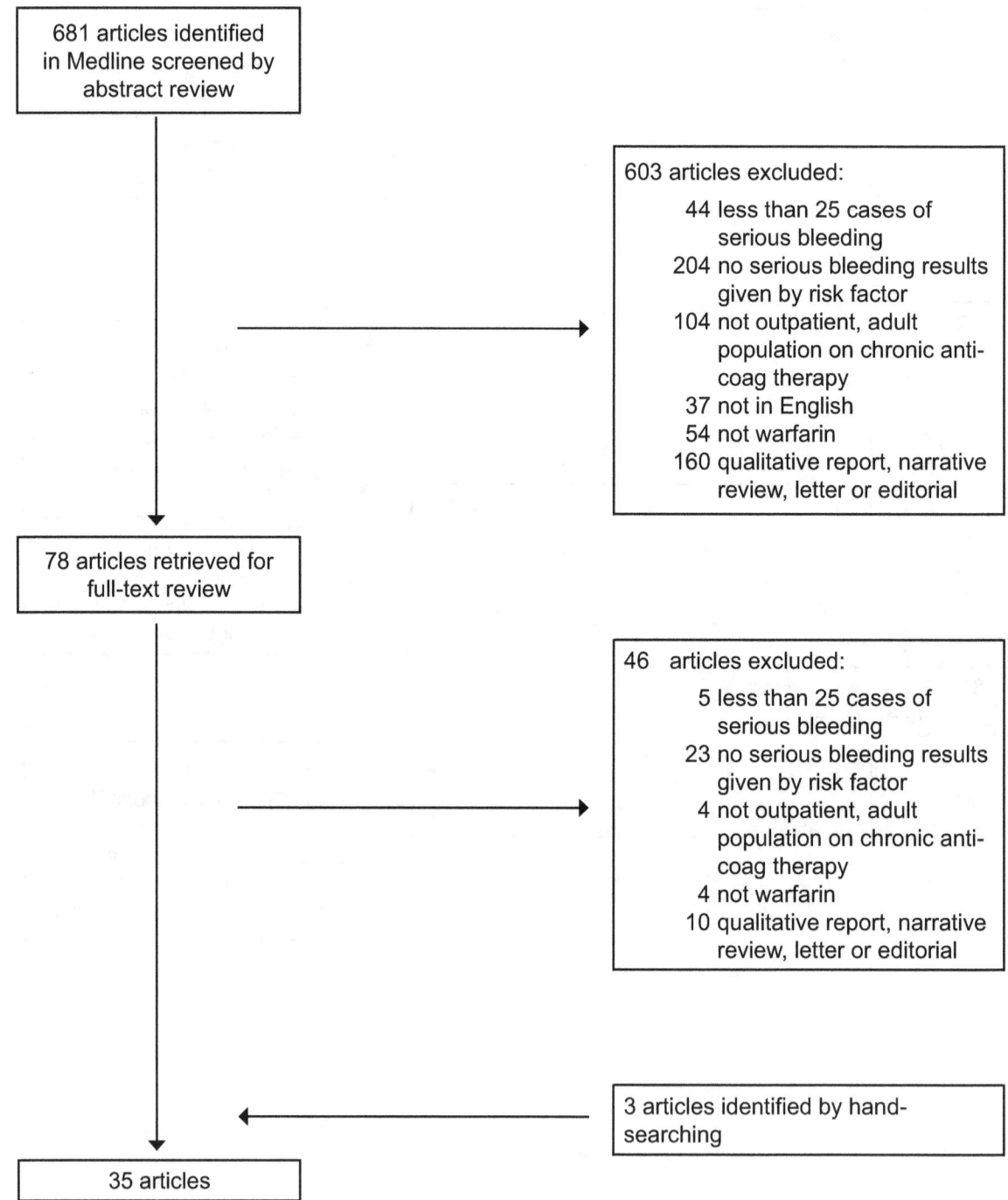

681 articles identified in Medline screened by abstract review

603 articles excluded:

- 44 less than 25 cases of serious bleeding
- 204 no serious bleeding results given by risk factor
- 104 not outpatient, adult population on chronic anti-coag therapy
- 37 not in English
- 54 not warfarin
- 160 qualitative report, narrative review, letter or editorial

78 articles retrieved for full-text review

46 articles excluded:

- 5 less than 25 cases of serious bleeding
- 23 no serious bleeding results given by risk factor
- 4 not outpatient, adult population on chronic anti-coag therapy
- 4 not warfarin
- 10 qualitative report, narrative review, letter or editorial

3 articles identified by hand-searching

35 articles

DATA EXTRACTION

For studies related to Key Questions 1 and 2, we extracted data on study design, country of origin, funding source, indications for anticoagulation, sample characteristics, interventions, mortality, thromboembolic events, major bleeding events, patient satisfaction, quality of life, laboratory measures of anticoagulation quality (i.e., percent time within the therapeutic range, percent of INR values within the therapeutic range, and INR variability), hospitalizations, outpatient and emergency room utilization, outpatient laboratory utilization, and long-term care admissions.

For Key Question #1a, we extracted data on ratio of staff to patient load; qualifications of staff and leadership; organizational structure of clinic; frequency and type (e.g., face-to-face versus phone) of contact with patient; frequency and timing of INR checks; use of computer-based algorithms to adjust dosing; timeliness of follow-up of abnormal INRs; patient education; use of genetic information to tailor therapy; protocols for use of vitamin K; clinic volume; hypercoagulation workups (e.g., Factor V Leiden); and use of technologies such as Interactive Voice Recording.

For Key Question #3, we extracted data on study characteristics, patient factors (e.g., age, gender, level of education); indication for anti-coagulation (atrial fibrillation; deep vein thrombosis/pulmonary embolism – either first or recurrent and with or without precipitating factors; mechanical heart valve; TIA/stroke; other); indices measuring severity of illness, functional status, and co-morbidity; time above therapeutic range; type of anticoagulant used; frequency and type of monitoring; concomitant use of anti-platelet agents; concomitant use of other medications; and setting within which patient is monitored (specialized anticoagulation clinic or not).

QUALITY ASSESSMENT

The quality of the individual randomized studies was assessed by the following: 1) adequate allocation concealment, denoted by central allocation, including telephone, web-based and pharmacy controlled randomization or use of sequentially numbered, opaque, sealed envelopes; 2) blinding of key study personnel (i.e., providers and/or study personnel who adjudicated outcomes blinded to group assignment); 3) analysis by intention-to-treat (i.e., all subjects counted in group to which they were randomized in the outcomes analyses); and 4) reporting of number of withdrawals/dropouts by group assignment.

DATA SYNTHESIS

For Key Question #1, analyses using a DerSimonian and Laird random-effects model, which assumes that the true treatment effects in the individual trials may vary from each other, were conducted in Review Manager Version 5.0.[3] A random-effects model is an analytical approach that incorporates heterogeneity that cannot be readily accounted for. Statistical heterogeneity between trials was assessed using the I^2 test. An I^2 score of 50 or greater indicates substantial heterogeneity.[4]

For Key Question #2, clinical outcomes data were pooled and analyzed in Review Manager

Version 5.0.[3] Because of low event rates for several clinical outcomes, we used Peto odds ratios (fixed effects model). Weighted mean differences were calculated using a random effects model using the Comprehensive Meta-Analysis software© (Biostat, Inc., Englewood, NJ). Statistical heterogeneity between trials was assessed using the I^2 test; a score of 50% or greater suggests moderate to substantial inconsistency among studies.[4] In order to explore heterogeneity we performed subgroup analyses and tested for interactions. The extent of publication bias was evaluated through visual inspection of funnel plot asymmetry and the linear regression–based test proposed by Egger.[5]

PEER REVIEW

A draft version of this report was sent to our Technical Expert Panel members and to three peer reviewers. Reviewer comments were addressed and our responses incorporated into the final report (Appendix A).

RESULTS

KEY QUESTION 1

For management of long-term outpatient anticoagulation in adults, are specialized anticoagulation clinics (ACC) more effective and safer than care in non-specialized clinics (e.g., primary care clinics, physician offices)?

Literature Search

Using the search strategy outlined in the Methods section, we searched for both randomized clinical trials and cohort studies published after 1996 in peer reviewed journals. We excluded non-English articles and studies that dealt with inpatients, pediatric populations, or short-term anticoagulation (< 3 months). As shown in Figure 2, we reviewed the abstracts of 612 articles of which 78 were selected for more detailed review. Of these, we identified a total of 10 articles. One more was obtained through a hand search for a total of 11 articles reporting on 3 randomized clinical trials and 8 cohort studies that met all inclusion criteria.

Randomized Controlled Trials

Overview of Included Studies (Table 1; Appendix B - Table 1)

The 3 trials were conducted in the US, China, and Canada. The Canadian trial randomized 221 subjects with mixed indications for outpatient anticoagulation (OAC) to either an ACC or usual care with a family physician and followed them for 3 months.[6] The Chinese trial randomized 138 subjects with mixed indications for OAC to either a hematologist-led or a pharmacist-led ACC and followed them for up to 2 years.[7] The US trial randomized practice clusters within 6 sites to either access or no access to an ACC; only subjects with atrial fibrillation as their indication for OAC were included.[8] Although 2 of the studies enrolled inception cohorts (i.e., patients new to anticoagulation), neither study was designed to detect differences in outcomes between the early and the maintenance anticoagulation phases.[6,7]

Subject Characteristics in the RCTs (Table 1)

A total of 722 subjects were enrolled in the 3 RCTs. The mean age of the subjects was 68 (range of study means, 59 to 76 years). Fifty one percent of subjects were male (range in studies, 45 to 58%). In the US study 37% of subjects were non-white;[8] in the Chinese study all subjects were Asian.[7] The Canadian study did not report race/ethnicity.[6] There were 359 patients in the 2 studies that allowed mixed indications for OAC[6,7] and 363 in the one study restricted to subjects with atrial fibrillation.[8]

Study Quality

The quality of the included studies was generally low. Only the Canadian study met all 4 of the quality indicators (adequate allocation concealment, some attempt at blinding, analyses by intention to treat [partially], and adequate description of study withdrawals).[6]

Interventions in the RCTs

In the US study,[8] the intervention consisted of an ACC which had responsibility for 3 core functions: management of anticoagulation which involved assigning patients to a medically qualified mid-level provider; screening administrative files to find eligible patients and offering ACC services to these patients' providers; and educating patients about anticoagulation.

In the Canadian study,[6] all enrolled patients received standard education regarding importance of medication compliance, self monitoring for clinical complications, dietary considerations, and possible medication interactions and were monitored by the ACC until they had achieved a stable dose of warfarin. They were then randomized to continued care in the ACC or with their primary care physician. Details of the procedures employed in the ACC were not included in the report.

In the Chinese study,[7] the intervention consisted of a pharmacist led clinic. The pharmacist received 1 month of training from 2 hematologists and was provided with a management protocol. A hematologist saw patients on their first visit to determine target INR range and duration of therapy. Patients in this arm received "intense education" during visits, written materials, and access to a pharmacist consultation through a telephone hotline.

Outcomes in the RCTs

The outcomes reported in each study are shown in Table 2. As shown in Table 3, there were very few major clinical outcome events and rates of all-cause mortality, major thromboembolic events, and major bleeding did not differ significantly between the two treatment arms in any of the 3 studies. Time within therapeutic range did not differ between intervention and control groups in the US and Canadian studies but was significantly higher in the intervention group in the Chinese study (64% v. 59%, p<0.05).

Two of the 3 RCTS evaluated patient satisfaction.[6,7] Using the Patient Satisfaction Questionnaire Short Form (PSQ-18), overall patient satisfaction was significantly higher in the intervention group (pharmacist managed) than in the control group (physician managed) (P <0.001).[7] Similar significant results were also found for the sub-scores measuring technical quality, interpersonal manner, communication, time spent with clinician and accessibility but there were no significant differences in the general satisfaction and financial sub-scores. In the second study,[6] patient satisfaction was measured by a "previously validated questionnaire", not referenced. Ninety six percent of patients in ACC reported being satisfied or very satisfied with their overall warfarin care compared with 84% of patients randomized to the family physician group (p=0.001). Specifically, patients in the ACC group reported significantly higher satisfaction with teaching, helpfulness of staff, availability of staff in an emergency, and time spent with staff than the subjects randomized to usual care.

In the one RCT that reported resource utilization,[7] there were no significant differences in cost per patient per month between the intervention and control groups for medication use, emergency room utilization, and hospitalizations.

Pooled Data

In the pooled analysis (Figure 5), there were 5 deaths in the ACC group and 6 in the Usual Care (UC) group, all from a single study (RR: 0.81, 95%CI: 0.25 to 2.58);[6] 6 major bleeding events in the ACC patients and 8 in UC patients (RR: 1.05, 95%CI: 0.36 to 3.12); 11 major thromboembolic events in the ACC and 14 in the UC patients (RR: 1.29, 95%CI: 0.59 to 2.81).

Laboratory Outcomes

Percent time in therapeutic range (TTR) by study group is shown in Table 4. In all 3 trials, %TTR was higher for the ACC than the UC group, but in only one was the difference statistically significant.[7] Overall, the pooled weighted mean of TTR for patients randomized to ACC was 59.9% (range of means 56-64%), only slightly higher than the 56.3% (range of means 52 to 59%) for the patients randomized to usual care, for a weighted mean difference of 3.6 (range of mean differences 3.3 to 5) (Table 5).

Cohort Studies

Overview of Included Studies (Table 1; Appendix B - Table 2)

Five of the 8 cohort studies were conducted in the US,[9-13] 1 in China,[14] 1 in Sweden,[15] and 1 in multiple countries.[16] Three studies were prospective[9,14,15] and 5 were retrospective cohort studies.[10-13,16] Five studies included subjects with mixed indications for OAC[9-12,15] and 3 included only subjects with atrial fibrillation.[13,14,16] One study enrolled an inception cohort, meaning that subjects had been on OAC for < 3 months,[10] 2 did not,[11,13] and in the other 5 it was unclear.[9,12,14-16] The one study that enrolled an inception cohort did not stratify outcomes by initiation vs. maintenance phases.[10] Follow-up was less than 12 months in 2,[9,12] 12 months in 2,[13,16] >12 months in 1,[15] and not reported in 3 studies.[10,11,14] In 4 studies, the intervention was an ACC run by a pharmacist,[9-12] in one it was an ACC run by a nurse,[13] in one it was defined as care provided in a systematic way by personnel focusing specifically on AC management,[16] and in 2 others the ACC was not described.[14,15]

Subject Characteristics in the Cohort Studies (Table 1)

A total of 12,768 subjects were included in the 8 observational studies. The mean age of subjects was 69 (range of study means, 57 to 74). Fifty five percent of subjects were male (range in studies 42 to 59%). Race/ethnicity was only reported in 2 studies. There were 9946 subjects in the studies that allowed mixed indications for OAC and 2822 in the 3 studies that restricted enrollment to atrial fibrillation.

Outcomes in the Cohort Studies

Reported outcomes are shown in Tables 2 and 3. In the only study in which all-cause mortality was reported, there were 3 deaths (0.09%) in the intervention group and 2 (0.06%) in the control group (p values not reported).[12] Four studies reported major thromboembolic events; in 1 of these the incidence was significantly higher in the control group,[10] in 1 it was significantly higher in the intervention group,[14] and in 2 studies p values were not reported.[12,13] The incidence of major bleeding events was significantly higher in the control group in 1 study,[10] and not significantly different between groups in 1 study.[14] Significance testing was not included for the 3 other studies that reported this outcome.[12,13,15] We were unable to pool major clinical outcomes because outcomes were reported as number of events in only 2 of the 8 studies;[12,14] the other studies reported events per patient- or treatment-year.

Laboratory Outcomes

As shown in Table 4, time within therapeutic range or percent of INR values within the therapeutic range was higher in the intervention group in all 6 studies that reported this metric.[10-14,16] As shown in Table 5, the weighted mean for percent time within therapeutic range for the 4 studies reporting this metric,[10,12,13,16] was 63.5% for the intervention groups and 53.5% for the control groups, for a difference of 10% (range of mean differences, 4.3 to 26%).

Other Outcomes

Three observational studies reported hospital admissions and/or emergency department (ED) visits.[9-11] In one there were no significant differences between UC and ACC groups for ED visits or inpatient admissions.[11] In the second,10 there were significantly fewer anticoagulation related hospitalizations (19 v 5) and ED visits (22 v 6) in the ACC group. For hospitalizations unrelated to AC use, there were no differences between the 2 groups but the group randomized to AC had significantly fewer ED visits for reasons deemed unrelated to anticoagulation. The third study,[9] reported warfarin-related hospital admissions in 10 control group patients vs. 3 ACC patients (p<0.01).

KEY QUESTION 1A

Which components of a specialized anticoagulation clinic are associated with effectiveness/ safety?

None of the included studies reported the **association** between **specific elements of ACC** (e.g. ratio of staff to patient load; qualifications of staff and leadership; organizational structure of clinic; frequency and type of contact with patient; use of computer-based algorithms to adjust dosing; patient education) and **outcomes**. In one RCT, patients in both arms received algorithm driven dose adjustments,[7] and in the other 2 studies only patients in the intervention arm were managed with dosing algorithms.[6,7] Among the 8 observational studies, 4 commented on possible processes of care that might have accounted for observed differences in outcomes. These included use of both face-to face and telephone interactions with patients,[13] use of a computerized patient monitoring system that identified patients who were delinquent in returning for timely INR determinations;[12] the specialized expertise of the ACC staff;[12] more consistency in ACCs in obtaining regular INRs;[11] and frequency of face-to-face consultations, methods of dosage adjustment, and provision of written dosage instructions.[16]

SUMMARY – KEY QUESTION 1

The evidence suggests that care provided within ACC may lead to better quality anticoagulation control as measured by time in therapeutic range but there is insufficient evidence to conclude that ACC care leads to fewer deaths, thromboembolic events, or major bleeding events than care provided in usual care settings such as primary care clinics. Patients were reported to like the convenience and enhanced service provided by these clinics.

Table 1. Summary of Study Characteristics for Anticoagulation Clinic versus Usual Care Studies (KQ1)

Characteristic	Randomized controlled trials (N=3)		Observational studies (N=8)	
	Range or Mean %	**# studies reporting**	**Range or Mean %**	**# studies reporting**
Overall: number of subjects per study	138 to 363 (722 total)	3	116 to 6645 (12,768 total)	8
Study dropouts/withdrawals, overall: mean % (range)	1 (0.7 to 1)	2	NA	NA
Age of subjects: mean years (range)	68 (59 to 76)	3	69 (57 to 74)	6
Gender, male: mean % (range)	51 (45 to 58)	3	55 (42 to 59)	8
Race/ethnicity, white: mean % (range)	45 (0 to 63)	2	73 (0 to 86)	2
Race/ethnicity, non-white: mean % (range)	55 (37 to 100*)	2	23 (14 to 100*)	2
Indication for anticoagulation, mixed indications:** number of subjects per study	138 to 221 (359 total)	2	116 to 6645 (9946 total)	5
Indication for anticoagulation, atrial fibrillation: number of subjects per study	363	1	204 to 1511 (2822 total)	3
Non-pharmacy, mixed (RN, NP, PA, PharmD, MD), or unclear managed anticoagulation clinic studies: number of subjects per study	221 to 363 (584 total)	2	204 to 2731 (5553 total)	4
Pharmacy-managed anticoagulation clinic studies: number of subjects per study	138	2	116 to 6645 (7215 total)	4†
Studies conducted in the United States: number of subjects per study	363	1	116 to 6645 (8322 total)	5
Prospective cohort studies: number of subjects per study	NA		136 to 2731 (3071 total)	3
Retrospective cohort studies: number of subjects per study			116 to 6645 (9697 total)	5

* 1 trial exclusively Asian

** Generally venous thromboembolism; CVA/stroke; heart valve replacement, atrial fibrillation, pulmonary embolus, myocardial infarction, cardiomyopathy or prophylaxis;

† All studies conducted in the United States

Table 2. Outcomes Reported for Anticoagulation Clinic versus Usual Care Studies (KQ1)

Study	Mortality	Thrombo-embolic events	Major bleeding events	Quality of life/patient satisfaction	% Time within therapeutic range	% INR values within therapeutic range	Emergency Room visits	Hospitaliza-tions
Randomized Trials								
Matchar 2002[8]		√	√		√			
Wilson 2003[6]	√	√	√	√	√			√
Chan 2006[7]	√	√	√	√	√		√	√
Observational Studies								
Lee 1996[9]								√
Chiquette 1998[10]		√	√		√	√	√	√
Chamberlain 2001[11]						√	√	√
Witt 2005[12]	√	√	√		√			
Du 2005[14]		√	√			√		
Ansell 2007[165]					√	√		
Wallvik 2007[15]			√					
Nichol 2008[13]		√	√		√			
TOTAL (11)	3	7	8	2	7	4	3	5

20

Table 3. Clinical Outcomes Events for Anticoagulation Clinic versus Usual Care Studies (KQ1)

Study	# All-cause deaths		# Thromboembolic events		# Major bleeding events	
	Intervention	Control	Intervention	Control	Intervention	Control
Randomized Trials						
Matchar 2002[8]			9/173 (5.2%)†	11/317 (3.5%)	3/173 (1.7%)†	5/317 (1.6%)
Wilson 2003[6]	5/112 (4.5%)†	6/109 (5.5%)	1/112 (0.9%)†	2/109 (1.8%)	2/112 (1.8%)†	1/109 (0.9%)
Chan 2006[7]	0/69†	0/69	1/68 (1.5%)†	1/69 (1.4%)	1/68 (1.5%)†	2/69 (2.9%)
Observational Studies						
Lee 1996[9]						
Chiquette 1998[10]			3.3% per pt-yr*	11.8% per pt-yr	9.7% per pt-yr*	39.2% per pt-yr*
Chamberlain 2001[11]						
Witt 2002[12]	3/3323 (0.09%)‡	2/3322 (0.06%)	17/3323 (0.5%)‡	41/3322 1.2%	29/3323 (0.9%)‡	31/3322 (0.9%)
Du 2005[14]			19/138 (13.8%)*	2/66 (3.0%)	8/138 (5.8%)†	2/66 (3.0%)
Ansell 2007[16]						
Wallvik 2007[15]					13/2292 tx-yrs‡	21/2752 tx-yrs
Nichol 2008[13]			1.9% per pt-yr‡	3.7% per pt-yr	2.3% per pt-yr‡	6.3% per pt-yr

* p<0.05
† Not statistically significant versus control
‡ p value not reported

Table 4. Laboratory Outcomes by Study Group for Anticoagulation Clinic versus Usual Care Studies

Study	% Time within therapeutic range		% INR values within therapeutic range		% Time above therapeutic range		% Time below therapeutic range	
	Intervention	Control	Intervention	Control	Intervention	Control	Intervention	Control
Randomized Trials								
Matchar 2002[8]	55.6%[†]	52.3%						
Wilson 2003[6]	63%[†]	59%						
Chan 2006[7]	64%[*]	59%						
Observational Studies								
Lee 1996[9]								
Chiquette 1998[10]	45.7%[*]	41.4%	36.6%[*]	31.3%				
Chamberlain 2001[11]			50.2%[‡]	45.8%				
Witt 2002[12]	63.5%[*]	55.2%	63.6%[*]	23.3%	11.8%[*]	14.5%	24.7%[*]	30.3%[*]
Du 2005[14]			63.6%[*]	23.3%				
Ansell 2007[16]	67[‡]	57.9%	59.1%[‡]	52%	13%	17%	20%	25%
Wallvik 2007[15]								
Nichol 2008[13]	68.1%[*]	42.1%			11.3%	9.4%	20.6%	48.5%

[*] p<0.05

[†] Not statistically significant versus control

[‡] p value not reported

Table 5. Weighted Means for the Percentage of Time within Therapeutic Range for Anticoagulation Clinic versus Usual Care Studies

Study	AC n	AC, % time within range	UC n	UC, % time within range	Mean difference
Randomized Trials					
Matchar 2002[8]	144	55.6%*	118	52.3%	3.3%
Wilson 2003[6]	112	63%*	106	59%	4%
Chan 2006[7]	68	64%**	69	59%	5%
Weighted means		59.9%		56.3%	Weighted mean difference = 3.6% (range of means 3.3 to 5)
Observational Studies					
Chiquette 1998[10]	176	45.7%**	142	41.4%	4.3%
Witt 2002[12]	3323	63.5%**	3322	55.2%	8.3%
Ansell 2007[16]	395	67%†	1116	57.9%	9.1%
Nichol 2008[13]	351	68.1%**	756	42.1%	26%
Weighted means		63.5%		53.5%	Weighted mean difference = 10% (range of means 4.3 to 26)

* Not statistically significant versus Usual Care

** p <0.05 versus Usual Care

† p value not reported

Figure 5. All-cause Mortality, Anticoagulation Clinic versus Usual Care

Study or Subgroup	Anticoagulation Clinic Events	Total	Usual Care Events	Total	Weight	Risk Ratio M-H, Random, 95% CI	Risk Ratio M-H, Random, 95% CI
Chan 2006 (7)	0	69	0	69		Not estimable	
Wilson 2003 (6)	5	112	6	109	100.0%	081 [0.25, 2.58]	
Total (95% CI)		**181**		**178**	**100.0%**	**0.81 [0.25, 2.58]**	
Total Events	5		6				

Heterogeneity, Not applicable

Test for overall effect: Z = 0.35 (P = 0.72)

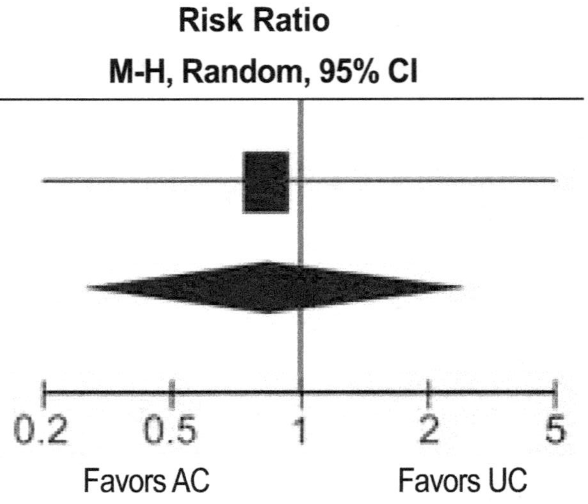

Favors AC Favors UC

0.2 0.5 1 2 5

KEY QUESTION 2

Is Patient Self Testing (PST), either alone or in combination with Patient Self Management (PSM), more effective and safer than standard care delivered in either ACCs or non-specialized clinics?

Literature Search

Using the search strategy shown in the Methods section, we looked for randomized clinical trials published after 1996 in peer reviewed journals. We excluded non-English articles as well as studies that dealt with inpatients, pediatric populations, or short-term anticoagulation (<3 months). As shown in Figure 3, we screened 2129 abstracts and selected 81 for full article review. Of these, we identified a total of 27 articles reporting on 22 distinct randomized clinical trials.

Overview of Included Studies

An overview of the 22 included studies is shown in Appendix B, Tables 3 and 4. Two studies were conducted in the US,[17,18] 1 in Canada,[19] and 19 in Europe.[20-45] Duration of follow-up was less than 12 months in 13 studies and 12 or more months in 9. A total of 8413 subjects were included in the 22 trials, with individual trial sample sizes ranging from 50 to 2922 (Table 6). Fourteen studies included patients with a variety of indications for anticoagulation[17-24,26,28-30,32,39-43] and 8 only included patients with mechanical heart valves (6)[31,33-38,44,45] or atrial fibrillation (2).[25,27] Three trials enrolled inception cohorts (i.e., limited enrollment to patients on OAC for < 3 months);[18,35-37,45] 11 trials did not enroll inception cohorts;[17,21-26,28-30,32,39,40,42,43] and in 8 studies the populations were either mixed or it was unclear.[19,20,27,31,33,34,38,41,44] Among the 3 with inception cohorts, outcomes were not analyzed by whether they had occurred in the anticoagulation initiation or maintenance phase.

Assessments of Quality and Bias

Measures of trial quality are shown in Figure 6 and reported in Appendix B, Tables 3 and 4. Allocation concealment was adequate in 9 trials, some attempt at blinding of endpoint assessors was made in 6, an intention to treat analysis was reported in 8, and number of drop-outs was reported in 18. Five trials met all 4 of these quality indicators.[17,20,24,41-43] Only six trials noted they received no funding from industry.[17,18,28,29,32,39] Egger's test suggested little evidence that small study effects influenced the findings for thromboembolic events (P = 0.513).

Subject Selection

The percentage of patients screened who met preliminary eligibility criteria, successfully completed the training, and agreed to be randomized was less than 20% in 4 studies,[22,23,30,45] between 20 and 50% in 7 studies,[24,25,28,32,39,41,43] and greater than 50% in 3 studies.[19,20] Eight studies did not report data; THINRS data is presented below. It is difficult to determine how many refusals were due to discomfort being in a trial vs. discomfort with self testing and/or self management of anticoagulation. Among patients who were randomized, the percentage who continued with the intervention throughout the study period ranged from 64-98%.

Subject Characteristics

The mean age of the subjects was 65 years (range of study means 42 to 75 years) (Table 6). Three studies specifically focused on elderly patients, enrolling only patients over the age of

65[18,25] or 60 years of age.[43] Seventy five percent of subjects were male (range in studies, 43 to 98%). Race/ethnicity was reported only in the 2 US studies, in one of those 8%[17] and in the other 33%[18] of the subjects were non-white. A total of 2911 subjects were enrolled in the 12 studies in which there were multiple indications for anticoagulation; 2074 were enrolled in the 6 studies restricted to a mechanical heart valve indication; 327 in the 2 studies limited to atrial fibrillation; and 3101 in the 2 trials that limited enrollment to mechanical heart valve or atrial fibrillation.

Interventions

Evaluated interventions included patient self testing only (i.e., dose adjustment made by the clinic, n=5)[17,18,25,32] and patient self-management (i.e. testing and dose adjustment made by patient, n=14).[19-22,25-28,30,31,35,36,38,39,41,43-45] In one study it was unclear if the intervention was PST or PSM.[34] In one study there were 4 arms (PST, PSM, routine care with or without education).[23] In one study there were 3 groups: routine care alone, routine care with education and PSM with education.[25] In one study PSM was compared to PST with no control group.[26,30] In 11 studies warfarin was used in all subjects,[17-19,22,25,26,30,32,38,39,44] other oral anticoagulants (phenprocoumon, acenocoumarol, fluindione) were used in 7,[20,21,23,31,35,36,41,43] in 3 studies the type of oral anticoagulant was not reported,[27,34,45] and in 1 study both warfarin and phenprocoumon were used.[28]

Details of PST/PSM Intervention:

The patient self testing/self management intervention usually included 2-4 small group training sessions of 1-3 hours over several weeks. The sessions, which were led by a nurse, pharmacist or physician, were followed by home practice and a test to ensure competency in all procedures. Training sessions typically included general information on anticoagulation, possible interactions with foods/medicines, how to use the INR testing machine (including demonstrating ability to use the machine correctly and to perform quality control checks), how to dose (usually by algorithm), how often to check INR, and when to call for help. Patients often had access to a 24 hour telephone help line. Two studies had much more intensive training. One of the US studies included one-on-one daily training by a lay educator while patients were still in the hospital followed by a home visit within 3 days of discharge.[18] The second study included a 24 week training program in which responsibility for dosing was gradually transferred from physician to patient,[28,29] A recent study from Ireland[32] employed an internet-based direct to patient expert system in which patients receive advice on dosing from the system after entering their INRs and relevant clinical information (e.g. intercurrent illnesses, dietary changes).

Control Intervention:

The control group received anticoagulation management in an ACC in 11 of the trials,[17,21-23,25,32,39,41,45] in a primary care or other physician office in 7 trials.[18-20,27,31,34-36,44] and in multiple settings in 3 trials.[28,38,42] The other trial compared PST to PSM without another control group.[26,30]

Outcomes

Reported outcomes are tabulated in Table 7 with details in Tables 8 and 9. All-cause mortality was reported in 16 studies, thromboembolic events in 20, major bleeding episodes in 20, and patient satisfaction and/or quality of life in 11. All studies reported one or more laboratory measure of quality of anticoagulation, the most common being a measure of time in therapeutic range in 18 studies.

Clinical Outcomes (Figures 7, 8, and 9)

There were 298 deaths in subjects randomized to PST/PSM intervention compared to 369 deaths in the control subjects (Peto OR: 0.74, 95%CI: 0.63 to 0.87, P=0.000), I²=51%). The intervention group had 283 major bleeding events compared with 300 in the control group (Peto OR: 0.89, 95%CI: 0.75 to 1.05, P=0.169, I²=2%). There were 99 major thromboembolic events in the intervention group compared with 149 in the control group (Peto OR 0.58, 95%CI: 0.45 to 0.75, P<0.000, I²=27%).

Sensitivity Analyses:

There was evidence of inconsistency among the studies, especially for the mortality outcome. In order to explore sources of heterogeneity we conducted subgroup analyses for all 3 clinical outcomes stratifying by the following variables: duration of study (<12 vs. ≥12 months), indication for anticoagulation (mechanical heart valve vs. all other), active intervention (PST vs. PSM), control intervention (ACC vs. physician office), study quality (met all 4 quality domains cited above), and funding source (industry vs. not reported vs. non-industry). Although in the initial analyses there were several significant interactions (i.e., for mortality: indication for anticoagulation, active intervention, control intervention, study quality, and funding source; for bleeding: study duration; and for thromboembolism: active intervention and funding source), only one remained marginally significant after we removed the VA trial, suggesting that the VA trial was a major contributing factor to the observed heterogeneity (see below for further discussion). The marginally significant interaction was for major bleeding by study duration (study duration: ≥ 12 months: Peto OR 1.04 95% CI 0.76 to 1.42; <12 months, Peto OR: 0.44, 0.22 to 0.85, P for interaction=0.02).

Effect of Patient Education on Outcomes:

Subjects enrolled in the PSM or PST arms of a trial receive more extensive training and education than patients assigned to usual care which might explain the difference in outcomes between the 2 groups. In the 2 studies that were designed to explore the independent effect of patient education, one found no effect of patient education on time in therapeutic range.[23,24] The other did find a significant effect on time in therapeutic range using a before-after within group comparison, rather than the more robust between group comparison.[25]

Outcome Differences between PST and PSM:

Two studies[23,30] compared PSM to PST. In neither study (Gadisseur[23] N=99 for this comparison; Gardiner[30] N =104) was there a significant difference in TTR between the 2 groups.

Percent Time in Therapeutic Range (TTR) by Study Group (Tables 9 and 10):

Overall, the pooled weighted mean of TTR for patients randomized to PST/PSM interventions was 66.1% (range of means 56-76.5%), only slightly higher than the 61.9% (range of means 32 to 77%) for the patients randomized to usual care (Table 10). As shown in Figure 10, for the studies we were able to include in a meta-analysis the weighted mean difference of 1.50% was not statistically significant (95% CI: -0.63 to 3.63%, I²=45%, 9 studies, P=0.168).

Percent of INRs within Therapeutic Range:

As shown in Tables 9 and 11, 11 studies reported mean values for this outcome. The pooled weighted mean was 70.5% (range of means 43 to 87%) in the PST/PSM group and 59.3% in the usual care group (range of means 22 to 78%). For the studies we were able to include in the meta-analysis, the weighted mean difference of 5.9% was not statistically significant (Figure 11) with a high level of heterogeneity (95%CI: -0.18 to 12.0%, I2=83%, 6 studies, P=0.057).

Patient Satisfaction and Quality of Life:

There is little uniformity in the measurement or definition of these constructs within the 11 studies that reported them.[17,19-,22,24-26,32,39,45] Three studies that used an instrument developed by Sawicki et al.[20] all found significant differences between the PST/PSM and the UC groups. Specifically, in the German study[20] patients randomized to PSM had significantly higher general treatment satisfaction and self efficacy, and significantly less distress and daily hassles than those in UC. In the cross-over study from the Netherlands,[21] patients in the self management group reported significantly more self-efficacy and general treatment satisfaction, and significantly less distress, social issues and daily worries than those in UC. In the third study, also from the Netherlands,[24] patients were randomized to usual care, PST only, and PSM. This study showed that patients in both intervention arms had significant reductions in daily hassles, distress, and strains in social network and increase in self efficacy and general satisfaction compared to the UC group. There were no statistically significant differences between the 2 intervention arms.

In 3 additional studies, one found that all of the patients who had been randomized to PSM wanted to continue the program after the study ended,[19] in the second, 77% indicated at the end of the study that they preferred self-testing to the hospital clinic,[26] and in the third, 98% expressed a preference for PST.[32] Three studies found no significant difference in patient satisfaction or quality of life between groups.[22,25,40] Patient satisfaction in the VA trial[17] is described below.

THINRS

This trial[17] is of particular interest since it was conducted in VA and is the largest trial to date comparing patient self-testing with usual care. The trial recruited 3,745 subjects in 28 VAMCs who required long term oral anticoagulation for either atrial fibrillation or a mechanical heart valve. Forty two of these subjects did not meet all entry criteria, 60 did not complete training, 586 did not undergo competency testing, 112 did not pass competency testing, and 23 passed the competency assessment but subsequently withdrew. Thus 78% of screened subjects were enrolled in the trial (N=2922). Subjects were randomized to high quality anticoagulation clinic management or patient self testing. Randomization was centralized and stratified by length of anticoagulation (< 3 months vs. ≥ 3 months) and indication. The primary endpoint was time to first event: stroke, major bleed, or death. Although the investigators and subjects were not blinded to treatment allocation, outcomes were assessed by independent adjudicators. An intention to treat analysis was performed. In both groups, loss to follow up was 1% in and warfarin discontinuation was 7%.

Ninety eight percent of the patients were male with a mean age of 67 (range of 33 to 99). Ninety two percent were white. Eighty three percent had atrial fibrillation and 24% had a mechanical heart valve. The primary endpoint was time to first event: stroke, major bleed, or death. The time to event curves did not differ significantly between intervention groups for either the primary endpoint or any of its three individual components. Time in target range and patient satisfaction were significantly higher in the PST group.

As indicated above, our results for major thromboembolism and bleeding appear to be robust with negligible heterogeneity, and similar findings have been reported in other reviews.[2,46,47] For mortality, however, there was evidence of inconsistency among studies that was likely attributable to the VA study. There are several possible reasons why the VA results differed from the other studies. First, this trial had substantially longer follow-up than any of the other studies and it may be that over time people assigned to PST stop testing as frequently leading to a lessening of the difference between those who are seen every month in the anticoagulation clinic and those who self test at home. Second, if the VA PST intervention was of lower quality than in other trials, this could explain its lower efficacy. However, this did not appear to be the case as the PST intervention included a rigorous patient education program and ongoing quality control which resulted in high percent time within therapeutic range. Finally, if the VA anticoagulation clinic was of higher quality than in the other trials, there would be less of an observed difference in outcomes between the 2 arms than in studies in which PSM/PST was compared to a lower quality control intervention. This likely was the case as the VA trial employed rigorous criteria to ensure that care in the anticoagulation clinics was state of the art.[17]

SUMMARY – KEY QUESTION 2

This review confirms that patient self testing with or without self management is at least as effective and safe as routine care for a select group of motivated adult patients requiring long term anticoagulation with Vitamin K antagonists.

Table 6. Summary of Study Characteristics for Patient Self Testing/Management versus Usual Care Studies

Characteristic	Range or Mean %	# studies reporting
Overall: number of subjects per study	50 to 2922 (8413 total)	22
Short-term trials (<12 months): number of subjects per study	50 to 341 (1935 total)	13
Long-term trials (≥12 months): number of subjects per study	62 to 2922 (6478 total)	9
Study dropouts/withdrawals, overall: mean % (range)	9 (<1 to 28)	18
Study dropouts/withdrawals, PST/PSM intervention: mean % (range)	14 (1 to 43)	15
Age of subjects: mean years (range)	65 (42 to 75)	19
Gender, male: mean % (range)	75 (43 to 98)	20
Race/ethnicity, white: mean % (range)	90 (67 to 92)	2*
Race/ethnicity, non-white/other: mean % (range)	10 (8 to 33)	
Indication for anticoagulation, mixed indications:* number of subjects per study	50 to 737 (3090 total)	13
Indication for anticoagulation, MHV replacement: number of subjects per study	62 to 930 (2074 total)	6
Indication for anticoagulation, atrial fibrillation: number of subjects per study	125 to 202 (327 total)	2
Indication for anticoagulation, MHV replacement and atrial fibrillation: number of subjects per study	2922	1
Studies conducted in the United States: number of subjects per study	325 to 2922 (3247 total)	2
Outcomes Assessed		
All-cause mortality: number of subjects per study	56 to 2922 (6820 total)	16
Event-related mortality: number of subjects per study	56 to 930 (3302 total)	9
Thromboembolic events: number of subjects per study	56 to 2922 (8209 total)	20
Major bleeding events: number of subjects per study	56 to 2922 (8209 total)	20
Percentage of time within therapeutic range: number of subjects per study	56 to 2922 (6008 total)	14
Percentage of INR within therapeutic range: number of subjects per study	50 to 765 (3857 total)	13
INR variability: number of subjects per study	67 to 765 (2268 total)	6

PST: patient self-testing; PSM: patient self-management; MHV: mechanical heart valve; INR: international normalized ratio
*Both studies conducted in the United States

Table 7. Outcomes Reported in Patient Self Testing/Management versus Usual Care Studies

Study	All-cause mortality	Event-related mortality	Thrombo-embolic events	Major bleeding events	Patient satisfaction & quality of life	% time within thera-peutic range	% INR values within thera-peutic range	INR variability	% time or INR values above or below range	No. of INR values	Cost-effective-ness
Short-term (<12 months) randomized, controlled trials											
Sawicki 1999[20]	✓		✓	✓	✓			✓			
Beyth 2000[18]	✓	✓	✓	✓		✓			✓	✓	
Cromheecke 2000[21]			✓	✓	✓	✓	✓	✓	✓		
Fitzmaurice 2002[22]	✓		✓	✓	✓	✓	✓			✓	✓
Gadisseur 2003 & 2004[23,24]			✓	✓	✓	✓	✓		✓	✓	
Khan 2004[25]			✓*	✓*	✓	✓		✓			
Sunderji 2004[19]	✓		✓	✓	✓	✓	✓		✓	✓	
Gardiner 2005[26]	✓		✓	✓	✓	✓					
Voller 2005[27]	✓		✓	✓		✓**	✓		✓	✓	
Christensen 2006 & 2007[28]	✓					✓		✓		✓	
Gardiner 2006[30]						✓				✓	
Dauphin 2008[31]	✓		✓	✓	✓	✓		✓			
Ryan 2009[32]			✓	✓	✓	✓	✓			✓	

Long-term (≥12 months) randomized, controlled trials

	16	6	20	20	11	18	12	8	9	13	3
Horstkotte 1996[33] & 1998[34]			√	√		√	√	√	√	√	
Koertke 2001[35,36] & 2007[37]	√	√	√	√		√	√		√	√	
Sidhu 2001[38]	√	√	√	√		√			√	√	
Fitzmaurice 2005[39] & Jowett 2006[40]	√	√	√	√	√	√					√
Menendez-Jandula 2005[41]	√	√	√	√		√	√	√		√	
Siebenhofer 2007[42] & 2008[43]	√	√	√	√		√	√	√	√	√	√
Eitz 2008[44]		√	√	√	√	√	√	√	√	√	
Soliman Hamad 2009[45]	√		√	√	√	√**	√				
Matchar 2010[17]	√		√	√	√	√					
TOTAL (20)	**16**	**6**	**20**	**20**	**11**	**18**	**12**	**8**	**9**	**13**	**3**

*only recorded in intervention groups **# of days (not % time)

Table 8. Clinical Outcomes Events for Patient Self Testing/Management versus Usual Care Studies

Study	All-cause mortality		Event-related mortality (# of deaths)		# Thromboembolic events		# Major bleeding events		Patient satisfaction & quality of life
	Intervention	Control	Intervention	Control	Intervention	Control	Intervention	Control	
Short-term (<12 months) randomized, controlled trials									
Sawicki 1999[20]	1/90 (1.1%)‡	1/89 (1.1%)	--	--	1/90 (1.1%)‡	2/89 (2.2%)	1/90 (1.1%)‡	1/89 (1.1%)	40-item questionnaire
Beyth 2000[18]	21/163 (13%)†	26/162 (16%)	1/163 (0.6%)‡	3/162 (1.8%)	14/163 (8.6%)†	21/162 (13.0%)	8/163 (4.9%)ˑ	17/162 (10.5%)	--
Cromheecke 2000[21]	--	--	--	--	0/50‡	1/50 (2%)	0/50	0/50	32-item questionnaire
Fitzmaurice 2002[22]	0/30‡	1/26 (3.8%)	0/30	1/26 (3.8%)	0/30	0/26	0/30‡	1/26 (3.8%)	Patient interview with SEIQoL tool
Gadisseur 2003[23] & 2004[24]	--	--	--	--	PST: 0/52 PSM: 0/47	P/Ed: 0/60 PC: 0/161	PST: 0/52 PSM: 2‡,a	P/Ed: 2‡,a PC: 1/161 (0.6%)	32-item questionnaire
Khan 2004[25]	1/44 (2.3%)‡	--	--	--	0/44	0/41	1/44 (2.3%)‡	0/41	Surveys with UKSF-36 and EuroQoL
Sunderji 2004[19]	0/70	0/70	0/70	0/70	0/70‡	2/70 (2.9%)	0/70‡	1/70 (1.4%)	--
Gardiner 2005[26]	1/44 (2.3%)‡	0/40	--	--	0/44	0/40	0/44	0/40	--
Voeller 2005[27]	0/101	0/101	0/101	0/101	0/101‡	1/101 (1%)	1/101 (1%)	0/101	--
Christensen 2006[28] & 2007[29]	1/50 (2%)	0/50	--	--	--	--	--	--	--
Gardiner 2006[30]	--	--	--	--	--	--	--	--	--
Dauphin 2008[31]	1/33 (3%)‡	0/34	--	--	0/33	0/34	0/33†	4/34 (11.8%)	--
Ryan 2009[32]	2 deaths, treatment arm not reported	--	--	--	2/132 (1.5%)	1/132 (0.8%)	0/132	1/132 (0.8%)	Patient satisfaction with care

Long-term (≥12 months) randomized, controlled trials

Study								
Horstkotte 1998[33,34]	---	---	---	---	0.9* (%/year)	3.63 (%/year)	4.49* (%/year)	10.88 (%/year)
Koertke 2001[35,36] & 2007[37]	At 5 years (est.) 32/447 (7.2%) At 12 years 94/488 (19.3%)‡	At 5 years (est.) 55/395 (13.9%) At 12 years 142/442 (32.2%)	8/488 (1.6%)‡	7/442 (1.6%)	16/579 (2.8%)*	32/576 (5.6%)	42/579 (7.3%)‡	34/576 (5.9%)
Sidhu 2001[38]	0/51†	4/49 (8.2%)	0/51	1/49 (2.0%)	1/51 (2.0%)‡	0/49	1/51 (2%)‡	0/49
Fitzmaurice 2005[39] & Jowett 2006[40]	5/337 (1.5%)‡	11/280 (3.9%)	2/337 (0.6%)‡	1/280 (0.4%)	4/337 (1.2%)‡	3/280 (1.1%)	5/337 (1.5%)‡	4/280 (1.4%)
Menendez-Jandula 2005[41]	6/368 (1.6%)‡	15/369 (4.1%)	3/368 (0.8%)‡	0/369	4/368 (1.1%)‡	20/369 (5.4%)	4/368‡ (1.1%)	7/369 (1.9%)
Siebenhofer 2007[42] & 2008[43]	15/99 (15.2%)†	11/96 (11.5%)	0/99†	3/96 (3.1%)	6/99 (6.1%)†	13/96 (13.5%)	7/99 (7.1%)	10/96 (10.4%)
Eitz 2008[44]	---	---	---	---	14/470 (3.0%)‡	21/295 (7.1%)	32/470‡ (6.8%)	20/295 (6.8%)
Soliman Hamad 2009[45]	1/29 (3.4%)	1/29 (3.4%)	---	---	0/29	1/29 (3.4%)	1/29 (3.4%)	1/29 (3.4%)
Matchar 2010[17]	152/1465 (10.4%)‡	157/1457 (10.8%)	---	---	33/1465 (2.3%)‡	31/1457 (2.1%)	180/1465 (12.3%)‡	199/1457 (13.7%)

Quality of life instrument column: Fitzmaurice 2005 & Jowett 2006 = "EQ-5D tool; mean QALYs"; Soliman Hamad 2009 = "SF-36v2"; all other studies = ---.

* p<0.05 versus control   † not statistically significant versus control   ‡ p value not reported   § range or deviation not reported
a quantity reported as events, not patients; we were therefore unable to determine a proportion since no denominator was available

CI = confidence interval   IQR = interquartile range (25-75%)   PC = primary care   PC/Ed = primary care with education   PSM = patient self-management
PST = patient self-testing   SD = standard deviation   SEM = standard error of the mean

Table 9. Laboratory Outcomes for Patient Self Testing/Management versus Usual Care Studies

Study	Mean % Time within therapeutic range		Mean % INR values within therapeutic range		INR variability (method)	
	Intervention	Control	Intervention	Control	Intervention	Control
Short-term (<12 months) randomized, controlled trials						
Sawicki 1999[20]	---	---	---	---	0.65±1.04* (mean squared INR deviation)	0.83±0.95
Beyth 2000[18]	56§	32	---	---	---	---
Cromheecke 2000[19]	---	---	55†,§	49	0.1±0.2‡ (mean difference)	0.12±0.22
Fitzmaurice 2002[22]	74‡ (95% CI 67-81)	77 (95% CI 67-86)	66‡ (95% CI 61-71)	72 (95% CI 65-80)	---	---
Gadisseur 2003[23] & 2004[24]	PST: 66.9† (95% CI 62.7-71) PSM: 68.6‡ (95% CI 63.7-73.6)	PC/Ed: 67.9 (95% CI 62.9-73) PC: 63.5 (95% CI 59.7-67.3)	PST: 63.9† (95% CI 59.8-68) PSM: 66.3† (95% CI 61-71.5)	PC/Ed: 61.3 (95% CI 55.4-67.1) PC: 58.7 (95% CI 55-62.4)	---	---
Khan 2004[25]	71.1‡ (SD 14.5)	PC/Ed: 70.4 (SD 24.5) PC: 63.2 (SD 25.9)	---	---	---	---
Sunderji 2004[19]	71.8† (SEM 5.5)	63.2 (SEM 5.8)	64.8† (SEM 5.8)	58.7 (SEM 5.9)	---	---
Gardiner 2005[36]	61‡ (SD 20, range 24-96)	64 (SD 26, range 7-100)	---	---	---	---
Voeller 2005[27]	---	---	67.8* (SD 17.6)	58.5 (SD 19.8)	---	---
Christensen 2006[28] & 2007[29]	78.7 (median)† (95% CI 69.2-81)	68.9 (median) (95% CI 59.3-78.2)	---	---	---	---

35

Study						
Gardiner 2006[30]	PST: 71.8[†] (95% CI 64.9-80.1, IQR 22.1) PSM: 69.9[†] (95% CI 60.8-76.7, IQR 23.1)	---	---	---	---	---
Dauphin 2008[31]	57[†] (SD 19)	53 (SD 19)	---	---	41.1±39.3[*] (mean deviation)	62.4±72.6
Ryan 2009[32]	74 (median) (p<0.001)	58.6 (median)	87.4	78.2	---	---
Long-term (≥12 months) randomized, controlled trials						
Horstkotte 1998[33,34]	---	---	43.2[‡,§]	22.3	---	---
Koertke 2001[35,36] & 2007[37]	---	---	78.3[*,§]	60.5	---	---
Sidhu 2001[38]	76.5[*,§]	63.8	---	---	---	---
Fitzmaurice 2005[39] & Jowett 2006[40]	70[†] (95% CI 68.1-72.4)	68 (95% CI 65.2-70.6)	---	---	---	---
Menendez-Jandula 2005[41]	64.3[†] (SD 14.3)	64.9 (SD 19.9)	58.6[*] (SD 14.3)	55.6 (SD 19.6)	0.58±0.18[†] (INR distance)	0.59±0.27
Siebenhofer 2007[42] & 2008[43]	73.4 (median) (IQR 64.7-82)	65.5 (median) (IQR 55.4-77.2)	68.4 (median)[*] (IQR 61.5-77.8)	59.1 (median) (IQR 50-70.6)	0.16[*] (IQR 0.09-0.25) (squared INR deviation)	0.23 (IQR 0.16-0.36)
Eitz 2008[44]	---	---	79[*,§]	65	0.35[*,§] (mean variance)	0.39
Soliman Hamad 2009[45]	---	---	72.9 (SD 11) (p=0.001)	53.9 (SD 14)	---	---
Matchar 2010[17]	**66.2 (SD 14.2)**	**62.4 (SD 17.1)**	---	---	---	---

* p<0.05   † p>0.05   ‡ p value not reported   § range or deviation not reported

CI = confidence interval   IQR = interquartile range (25-75%)   PC = primary care   PC/Ed = primary care with education
PSM = patient self-management   PST = patient self-testing   SD = standard deviation   SEM = standard error of the mean

Table 10. Percentage of Time within Therapeutic Range for Patient Self Testing/Management versus Usual Care Studies*

Study	PST/PSM group	Standard care group
Short-term studies (<12 months)		
Beyth 2000[18] (n=325)	56	32
Fitzmaurice 2002[22] (n=49)	74	77
Gladisseur 2003[23] (n=320)	*PST* 66.9	*PC/Ed*** 67.9
	PSM 68.6	*PC* 63.5
Khan 2004[25] (n=79)	71.1	70.4
Sunderji 2004[19] (n=139)	71.8	63.2
Gardiner 2005[26] (n=88)	61	64
Dauphin 2008[31] (n=67)	57	53
Long-term studies (≥12 months)		
Sidhu 2001[38] (n=84)	76.5	63.8
Fitzmaurice 2005[39] (n=617)	70	68
Menedez-Jandula 2005[41] (n=737)	64.3	64.9
Matchar 2010[17] (n=2870)	66.2	62.4
Pooled weighted mean (range)	**66.1 (56 to 76.5)**	**61.9 (32 to 77)**

*Includes only studies that reported *mean* percentage of time
**PC = primary care; PC/Ed = primary care with education

Table 11. Percentage of INR Values within Therapeutic Range for Patient Self Testing/Management versus Usual Care Studies*

Study	PST/PSM group	Standard care group
Short-term studies (<12 months)		
Cromheecke 2000[21] (n=50)	55	49
Fitzmaurice 2002[22] (n=49)	66	72
Gladisseur 2003[23] (n=320)	*PST* 63.9	*PC/Ed*** 61.3
	PSM 66.3	*PC* 58.7
Sunderji 2004[19] (n=139)	64.8	58.7
Voeller 2005[27] (n=202)	67.8	58.5
Ryan 2009[32] (n=132)	87.4***	78.2***
Long-term studies (≥12 months)		
Horstkotte 1998[34] (n=150)	43.2	22.3
Koertke 2001[35,36] (n=575)	78.3	60.5
Menedez-Jandula 2005[41] (n=737)	58.6	55.6
Eitz 2008[44] (n=765)	79	65
Soliman Hamad 2009[45] (n=62)	72.9	53.9
Pooled weighted mean (range)	**70.5 (43.2 to 87.4)**	**59.3 (22.3 to 78.2)**

*Includes only studies that reported *mean* percentage of values
**PC = primary care; PC/Ed = primary care with education
***Within 0.75 units of INR of the target INR

Figure 6. Methodological Quality Summary, Patient Self Testing/Management Studies <u>versus Usual Care Studies</u>

	Allocation concealment?	Blinding (outcomes assessors or evaluation of dosing)	Intention-to-treat	Withdrawals described
Beyth 2000 (18)		+		+
Christensen 06/07 (28,29)	−	−	−	+
Cromheecke 2000 (21)	+			+
Dauphin 2008 (31)		−		+
Eitz 2008 (44)			−	−
Fitzmaurice 2002 (22)		−	−	+
Fitzmaurice 2005 (26)	+	−	+	+
Gadisseur 2004 (24)	+	+	+	+
Gardiner 2005 (26)		−		+
Gardiner 2006 (30)		−		
Horstkotte 1998 (34)				
Khan 2004 (40)			−	+
Koertke 2001/07 (35,36)				+
Matchar 2010 (17)	+	+	+	+
Menendez-J 2005 (41)	+	+	+	+
Ryan 2009 (32)	+	−	−	+
Sawicki 1999 (20)	+	+	+	+
Sidhu 2001 (38)				+
Siebenhofer 07/08 (42,43)	+	+	+	+
Soliman Hamad 2009 (45)		−	−	
Sunderji 2004 (19)		−	+	+
Voller 2005 (27)		−		

Figure 7. All-cause Mortality, Patient Self Testing/Management versus Usual Care Studies

Study or Subgroup	Patient Self-Testing/Management Events	Total	Usual Care Events	Total	Weight	Peto Odds Ratio Peto, Fixed, 95% CI	Peto Odds Ratio Peto, Fixed, 95% CI
2.1.1 Short-term trials (<12 months)							
Beyth 2000 (18)	21	163	26	162	7.2%	0.77 [0.42, 1.44]	
Christensen 2007 (29)	1	50	0	50	0.2%	7.39 [0.15, 372.38]	
Dauphin 2008 (31)	1	33	0	34	0.2%	7.62 [0.15, 384.01]	
Fitzmaurice 2002 (22)	0	30	1	26	0.2%	0.12 [0.00, 5.91]	
Gardiner 2005 (26)	1	44	0	40	0.2%	6.75 [0.13, 341.54]	
Sawicki 1999 (20)	1	90	1	89	0.4%	0.99 [0.06, 15.93]	
Sunderji 2004 (19)	0	70	0	70		Not estimable	
Voller 2005 (27)	0	101	0	101		Not estimable	
Subtotal (95% CI)		581		572	8.2%	0.87 [0.49, 1.55]	
Total events	25		28				
Heterogeneity: Chi² = 4.52, df = 5 (P = 0.48); I² = 0%							
Test for overall effect: Z = 0.48 (P = 0.63)							
2.1.2 Long-term trials (≥12 months)							
Fitzmaurice 2005 (39)	5	337	11	280	2.7%	0.38 [0.14, 1.03]	
Koertke 2007 (37)	94	488	142	442	31.2%	0.51 [0.38, 0.68]	
Matchar 2010 (17)	152	1465	157	1457	49.1%	0.96 [0.76, 1.21]	
Menendez-Jand. 2005 (41)	6	368	15	369	3.6%	0.42 [0.17, 0.99]	
Sidhu 2001 (38)	0	51	4	49	0.7%	0.12 [0.02, 0.89]	
Siebenhofer 2008 (43)	15	99	11	96	4.0%	1.37 [0.60, 3.13]	
Soliman Hamad 2009 (45)	1	29	1	29	0.3%	1.00 [0.06, 16.39]	
Subtotal (95% CI)		2837		2722	91.8%	0.73 [0.61, 0.86]	
Total events	273		341				
Heterogeneity: Chi² = 19.63, df = 6 (P = 0.003); I² = 69%							
Test for overall effect: Z = 3.63 (P = 0.0003)							
Total (95% CI)		3418		3294	100.0%	0.74 [0.63, 0.87]	
Total events	298		369				
Heterogeneity: Chi² = 24.49, df = 12 (P = 0.02); I² = 51%							
Test for overall effect: Z = 3.61 (P = 0.0003)							
Test for subgroup differences: Chi² = 0.34, df = 1 (P = 0.56), I² = 0%							

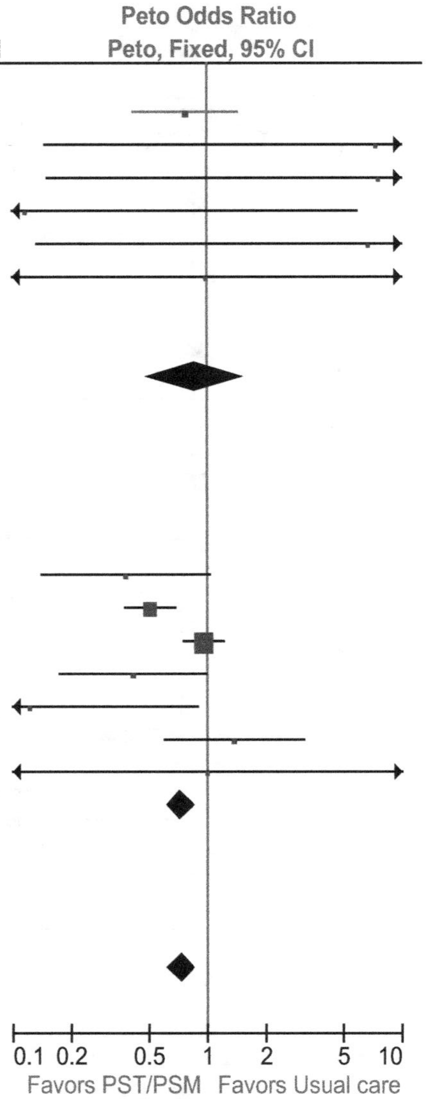

Favors PST/PSM   Favors Usual care

Figure 8. Major Bleeding Events, Patient Self Testing/Management versus Usual Care Studies

Study or Subgroup	Patient Self-Testing/Management Events	Total	Usual Care Events	Total	Weight	Peto Odds Ratio Peto, Fixed, 95% CI
2.2.1 Short-term trials (<12 months)						
Beyth 2000 (18)	8	163	17	162	4.5%	0.46 [0.20, 1.03]
Cromheecke 2000 (21)	0	50	0	50		Not estimable
Dauphin 2008 (31)	0	33	4	34	0.7%	0.13 [0.02, 0.94]
Fitzmaurice 2002 (22)	0	30	1	26	0.2%	0.12 [0.00, 5.91]
Gardiner 2005 (26)	0	44	0	40		Not estimable
Khan 2004 (25)	1	44	0	41	0.2%	6.90 [0.14, 348.69]
Ryan 2009 (32)	0	132	1	132	0.2%	0.14 [0.00, 6.82]
Sawicki 1999 (20)	1	90	1	89	0.4%	0.99 [0.06, 15.93]
Sunderji 2004 (19)	0	70	1	70	0.2%	0.14 [0.00, 6.82]
Voller 2005 (27)	1	101	0	101	0.2%	7.39 [0.15, 372.38]
Subtotal (95% CI)		663		655	6.5%	0.43 [0.22, 0.85]
Total events	11		25			

Heterogeneity: Chi² = 6.83, df = 7 (P = 0.45); I² = 0%
Test for overall effect: Z = 2.43 (P = 0.02)

Study or Subgroup	Events	Total	Events	Total	Weight	Peto Odds Ratio
2.2.2 Long-term trials (≥12 months)						
Eitz 2008 (44)	32	470	20	295	8.9%	1.00 [0.56, 1.79]
Fitzmaurice 2005 (39)	5	337	4	280	1.7%	1.04 [0.28, 3.89]
Koertke 2001 (35,36)	42	579	34	576	13.7%	1.25 [0.78, 1.98]
Matchar 2010 (17)	180	1465	199	1457	63.6%	0.89 [0.71, 1.10]
Menendez-Jand. 2005 (41)	4	368	7	369	2.1%	0.58 [0.18, 1.90]
Sidhu 2001 (38)	1	51	0	49	0.2%	7.10 [0.14, 358.35]
Siebenhofer 2008 (43)	7	99	10	96	3.0%	0.66 [0.24, 1.78]
Soliman Hamad 2009 (45)	1	29	1	29	0.4%	1.00 [0.06, 16.39]
Subtotal (95% CI)		3398		3151	93.5%	0.93 [0.78, 1.11]
Total events	272		275			

Heterogeneity: Chi² = 3.93, df = 7 (P = 0.79); I² = 0%
Test for overall effect: Z = 0.78 (P = 0.43)

Total (95% CI)		4061		3806	100.0%	0.89 [0.75, 1.05]
Total events	283		300			

Heterogeneity: Chi² = 15.36, df = 15 (P = 0.43); I² = 2%
Test for overall effect: Z = 1.38 (P = 0.17)
Test for subgroup differences: Chi² = 4.60, df = 1 (P = 0.03), I² = 78.3%

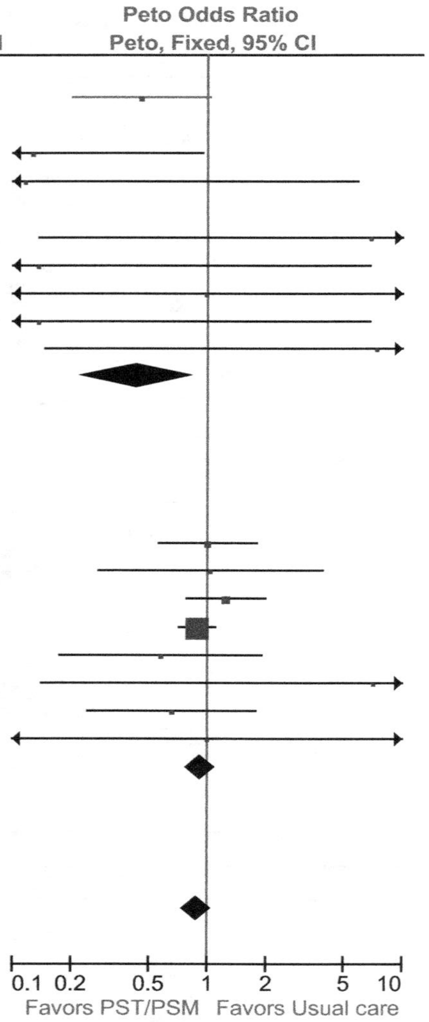

Peto Odds Ratio Peto, Fixed, 95% CI

0.1 0.2 0.5 1 2 5 10

Favors PST/PSM   Favors Usual care

Figure 9. Major Thromboembolic Events, Patient Self Testing/Management versus Usual Care Studies

Study or Subgroup	Patient Self-Testing/Management Events	Total	Usual Care Events	Total	Weight	Peto Odds Ratio Peto, Fixed, 95% CI	Peto Odds Ratio Peto, Fixed, 95% CI
2.3.1 Short-term trials (<12 months)							
Beyth 2000 (18)	14	163	21	162	13.6%	0.64 [0.32, 1.28]	
Cromheecke 2000 (21)	0	50	1	50	0.4%	0.14 [0.00, 6.82]	
Dauphin 2008 (31)	0	33	0	34		Not estimable	
Fitzmaurice 2002 (22)	0	30	0	26		Not estimable	
Gadisseur 2003 (23)	0	99	0	221		Not estimable	
Gardiner 2005 (26)	0	44	0	40		Not estimable	
Khan 2004 (25)	0	44	0	41		Not estimable	
Ryan 2009 (32)	2	132	1	132	1.3%	1.96 [0.20, 18.98]	
Sawicki 1999 (20)	1	90	2	89	1.3%	0.50 [0.05, 4.91]	
Sunderji 2004 (19)	0	70	2	70	0.9%	0.13 [0.01, 2.15]	
Voller 2005 (27)	0	101	1	101	0.4%	0.14 [0.00, 6.82]	
Subtotal (95% CI)		856		966	17.9%	0.58 [0.32, 1.07]	
Total events	17		28				
Heterogeneity: Chi² = 3.31, df = 5 (P = 0.65); I² = 0%							
Test for overall effect: Z = 1.73 (P = 0.08)							
2.3.2 Long-term trials (≥12 months)							
Eitz 2008 (44)	14	470	21	295	13.7%	0.39 [0.19, 0.78]	
Fitzmaurice 2005 (39)	4	337	3	280	3.0%	1.11 [0.25, 4.94]	
Koertke 2001 (35,36)	16	579	32	576	19.9%	0.50 [0.28, 0.88]	
Matchar 2010 (17)	33	1465	31	1457	27.1%	1.06 [0.65, 1.74]	
Menendez-Jand. 2005 (41)	4	368	20	369	10.1%	0.25 [0.11, 0.57]	
Sidhu 2001 (38)	1	51	0	49	0.4%	7.10 [0.14, 358.35]	
Siebenhofer 2008 (43)	6	99	13	96	7.5%	0.43 [0.17, 1.10]	
Soliman Hamad 2009 (45)	0	29	1	29	0.4%	0.14 [0.00, 6.82]	
Subtotal (95% CI)		3398		3151	82.1%	0.58 [0.43, 0.77]	
Total events	78		121				
Heterogeneity: Chi² = 14.46, df = 7 (P = 0.04); I² = 52%							
Test for overall effect: Z = 3.79 (P = 0.0001)							
Total (95% CI)		4254		4117	100.0%	0.58 [0.45, 0.75]	
Total events	95		149				
Heterogeneity: Chi² = 17.77, df = 13 (P = 0.17); I² = 27%							
Test for overall effect: Z = 4.17 (P < 0.0001)							
Test for subgroup differences: Chi² = 0.00, df = 1 (P = 0.97), I² = 0%							

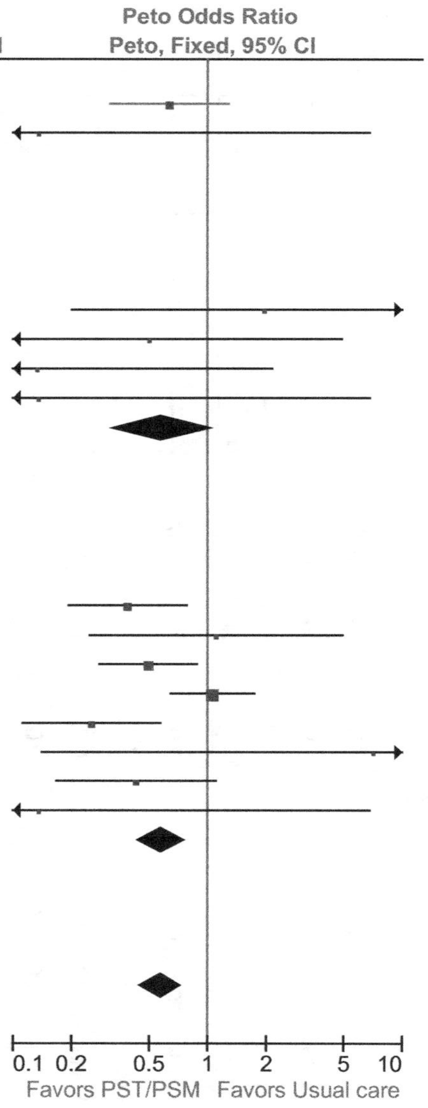

Plot axis: 0.1 0.2   0.5   1   2   5   10   Favors PST/PSM   Favors Usual care

Figure 10. Percent Time in Therapeutic Range for Patient Self Testing/Management versus Usual Care Studies

Study name	Difference in means	Lower limit	Upper limit
Fitzmaurice 2002 (22)	-3.00	-14.45	8.45
Gadisseur 2003 (23)	-1.00	-7.54	5.54
Sunderji 2004 (19)	8.60	-7.07	24.27
Khan 2004 (25)	0.70	-8.15	9.55
Gardiner 2005 (26)	-3.00	-12.87	6.87
Dauphin 2008 (31)	4.00	-5.10	13.10
Menendez-J 2005 (41)	-0.60	-3.10	1.90
Fitzmaurice 2005 (39)	2.00	-1.41	5.41
Matchar 2010 (17)	3.80	2.65	4.95
	1.50	-0.63	3.63

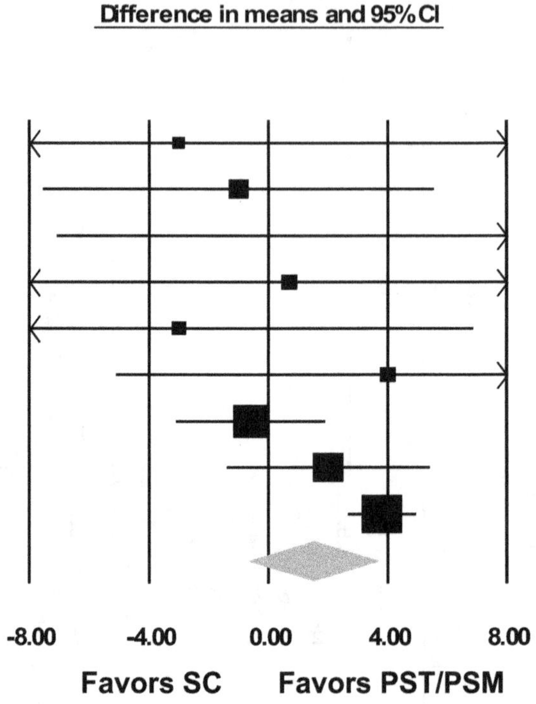

Difference in means and 95% CI. -8.00 -4.00 0.00 4.00 8.00. Favors SC   Favors PST/PSM

Figure 11. Percent of INRs within Therapeutic Range for Patient Self Testing/Management versus Usual Care Studies

Study name	Difference in means	Lower limit	Upper limit
Fitzmaurice 2002 (22)	-6.00	-14.82	2.82
Gadisseur 2003 (23)	2.60	-4.62	9.82
Sunderji 2004 (19)	6.10	-10.13	22.33
Voller 2005 (27)	9.30	4.13	14.47
Menendez-J 2005 (41)	3.00	0.52	5.48
Soliman Hamad 2009 (45)	19.00	12.52	25.48
	5.91	-0.18	12.01

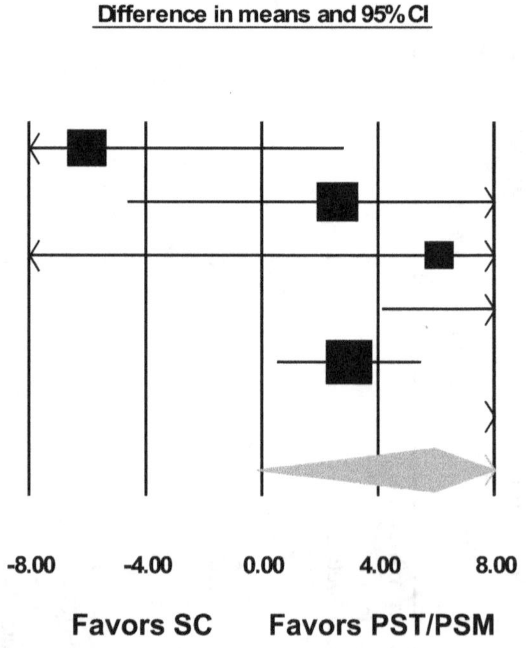

Difference in means and 95% CI. -8.00 -4.00 0.00 4.00 8.00. Favors SC   Favors PST/PSM

KEY QUESTION 3

What are the risk factors for serious bleeding in patients on chronic anticoagulant therapy?

Literature Search

Using the search strategy shown in the Methods section, we looked for studies published in English after 1996 in peer reviewed journals. We included studies that provided rates of serious bleeding events in populations who were on warfarin therapy. The rates of serious bleeding needed to either be presented by strata of risk factors (e.g., 1% in people less than 50 years and 1.4% in people over 50 years of age) or using a ratio of risk such as an odds ratio, relative risk or hazards ratio (e.g., HR=1.4 for people over age 50 compared to people under age 50). We excluded studies that did not report at least 25 cases of serious bleeding, since the precision for estimated risk among small studies is limited and observational studies such as those identified in this report are too heterogeneous to pool for formal meta-analysis. We excluded reports that dealt with inpatients, pediatric populations, or non-warfarin anticoagulation. As shown in Figure 4, we screened 681 titles/abstracts and selected 78 for full article review. Of these, we identified a total of 32 articles reporting on 33 distinct studies.[48-79] We also identified three additional articles by hand-searching references cited.[80-82]

Overview of Included Studies

An overview of the 35 included articles is shown in Appendix B, Table 5. These 35 articles represent 35 unique studies (several studies were reported in multiple articles, 1 article included a development and validation cohort, a series of articles reported on the warfarin arm of two randomized controlled trials, and 1 article reported a meta-analysis of 6 randomized trials). There were three multinational studies, 17 US studies (including 3 studies with a substantial VA population). Study designs included: meta-analyses, RCTs of additional drugs combined with warfarin, warfarin arms of RCTs analyzed as prospective cohort studies, observational retrospective/prospective cohort studies, case-control studies, and case-control studies nested in cohort studies. Within these different study designs various analytical methods were used, ranging from simply reporting frequencies of serious bleeding events by strata of a risk factor to using multivariable models to estimate the independent effect of a risk factor after accounting for many other potential risk factors and follow-up time. Average follow-up times ranged from slightly less than a year to 5 years, with most studies reporting follow-up periods of 1 to 2 years.

Subject Characteristics

A total of 453,918 subjects were included in these studies. Studies ranged in size from a case control study with 26 cases and 56 controls to a large administrative database study of Medicare records that included 353,489 patients. Since any averages of patient characteristics by study will be mostly driven by the few large administrative studies, the value of overall patient characteristics is somewhat limited. Most studies included primarily elderly populations with an average age of approximately 70 years. The distribution of gender represented in the studies varied widely with a maximum of 98.5% male to a minimum of 23% male.

Predictors of Serious Bleeding

Of the 35 articles we identified that provided evidence regarding the impact of various risk factors for predicting serious bleeding events, each article provided a different set of reported risk factors in a diverse range of patient populations, using different lengths of follow-up. These differences make statistical pooling of results unreliable, so the evidence is summarized below in a narrative format. All of the quantitative results extracted from the 35 studies are presented in Appendix B, Table 5. The risk factors reported in each study are displayed in Table 12.

Age

Overall, there is evidence that older age is associated with increased risk of serious bleeding in patients on warfarin. The evidence is not completely consistent across studies and also tends to suggest that the association is not linear in that the difference in risk between a 40 and 60 year old is likely not the same as the difference in risk between a 60 and 80 year old.

Sixteen articles from 14 unique studies reported results regarding the impact of increased age on the risk of serious bleeding events in people on warfarin therapy.[48-52,58,61,62,63,65,66,72,74,76,77,79] Increased age was typically found to be associated with increased bleeding risk;[48,48,51,58,62,63,66,76,77,79] however several studies failed to show a significant association between increased age and increased risk of serious bleeding events.[50,52,61,72,74] Furthermore, in the studies that did show a significant age association, the magnitude of the association differed substantially between studies. The amount of increased bleeding attributable to increased age ranged from a few studies reporting several fold higher rates of bleeding events in the oldest age groups (i.e., those over 80) compared to people in their 50s to 60s, while most other studies reported more modest to completely null associations. This suggests that the association between patient age and bleeding is likely complex and dependent on other factors that act as either confounders or effect modifiers. Another difference between studies related to the format in which age was modeled. In some studies results were reported from multivariable adjusted models based estimates of a one year increase in age, while others used dichotomous comparisons of differences above and below an age cut point (e.g., above versus below age 65). Still others simply reported unadjusted rates of bleeding across several age categories.

Gender

Overall, in the studies we identified, gender was not strongly associated with the rate of serious bleeding. Only nine articles reported results regarding the impact of gender on the risk of serious bleeding events in people on warfarin therapy.[48,50,52,59,61,65,66,72,77] Among the studies that reported results by gender, most failed to observe a significant association between gender and risk of serious bleeding.[48,52,59,61,65,77] In a large U.S. study using administrative data, men and women had similar rates of overall hemorrhage (RR: 1.25, 95%CI; 0.91–1.67), but men had a two-fold risk of intracranial hemorrhage (RR: 2.0, 95%CI; 1.11–3.33).[59] Likewise data from two large trials show that the rate of major bleeding on warfarin was not significantly different between men and women (p=0.49) with men having 0.35% more events per year (a non-significant relative difference of approximately 14%).[65] One study from Sweden found men had a 2.8 fold higher rate of severe hemorrhage (95%CI: 1.1-7.3).[72] Conversely, one U.S. study identified a small, but statistically significant increased risk of major bleeding in women.[66] This study was used to develop the bleeding risk index (mentioned below), and this is the one index that incorporates female gender as a predictor of bleeding risk.

Aspirin, NSAIDs, and other Medication Use

Aspirin use has been associated with increased risk of bleeding in patients on warfarin and the relative increase in risk is likely greater than two-fold. Aspirin is the only predictor we investigated for which we identified evidence from randomized controlled trials. A meta-analysis of six RCTs including 3,874 participants, in which 31 cases of intracranial hemorrhage developed, showed a 2.4 fold increased risk (95%CI; 1.2-4.8) among those randomized to aspirin plus warfarin compared to those randomized to only warfarin.[53]

When data are available from randomized trials the value of nonrandomized data is reduced. This is particularly true for drugs where confounding by indication can occur, such that it is difficult to untangle whether it is the drug or the indication for taking the drug that might predispose someone to a higher risk of events. Data from studies that did not randomize patients to aspirin but still compared rates of bleeding by reported aspirin use have also consistently reported increased bleeding in those taking aspirin and the increase has tended to be close to a doubling of the risk of serious bleeding events.[58,60,62,64,70]

The evidence for an increased risk of serious bleeding is not as strong for other medications. NSAIDs have been reported, from observational studies, to be associated with increased risks of serious bleeding events, but these risks are generally weaker in magnitude (less than two-fold increased risk) and less consistently reported than the results from studies of aspirin.[45,52,57,74] We found no randomized controlled trials confirming the association of NSAIDs with serious bleeding events.

In the studies we identified, few other medications were regularly reported with serious bleeding outcomes. A study by Gasse et al. listed several medications which were associated with increased risks of bleeding among patients taking their first ever dose of warfarin.[60] Several medications were associated with increased risk of bleeding some of which were associated with very high risks of bleeding (see Appendix B, Table 5), but most of these medications were either not reported or not assessed in the other studies we identified.

Warfarin Duration

Serious bleeding events tend to occur most frequently during the initiation of warfarin therapy.[51,62,63,72] Among the studies that reported the rate of serious bleeding by the duration of time on warfarin, the most commonly reported first interval was events at 1 month and then typically the rate at 12 months and possibly later was also reported. Only one study reported similar rates of bleeding events during the first month compared to all other months.[74] This same study also found no difference in bleeding rates between new users and chronic warfarin users. All four of the studies showed initial bleeding rates that were two to three times higher in the first one to three months compared to the rest of follow-up. The absolute magnitude of bleeding during the first month varied substantially in magnitude possibly due to differences in the study population and definition of serious bleeding. However there was a clear trend for decreasing rate of bleeding events after the initial few months of warfarin treatment.

INR — We identified only two studies that reported serious bleeding events by INR variability.[81,82] Both studies reported that increased INR variability was associated with an increase in the risk of serious bleeding. However, in one study the impact of INR variability was only seen among people who spent the greatest amount of time outside of the INR target range of 2.5-4.0.[82]

Primary Indication

We identified only two studies that reported serious bleeding events by the primary indication for taking warfarin.[50,74] Both studies reported that patients taking warfarin because of valve conditions were at significantly increased risk of bleeding compared to other patients. While this may have little impact for patient care since it is not modifiable, it is a relevant factor to consider when evaluating the overall bleeding risk of a population on warfarin.

Genetic Factors

Several recent articles have attempted to predict risk of serious bleeding events using genetic polymorphisms in two genes (CYP2C9 and VKORC1).[54,71,73] These articles represent two unique studies including approximately 631 patients and 75 cases of serious bleeding. Both studies reported participants with variant CYP2C9 genotypes having a roughly three-fold greater rate of serious bleeding events compared to those with the CYP2C9 wild type genotype.[54,71,73] The association between the VKORC1 genotypes and serious bleeding was not significant in either study.[71,73]

Co-morbidity

Twelve studies reported on various co-morbidities and their associations with increased risk of serious bleeding events.[48,50,51,52,55,57,61,62,66,75,79,81] There was not a consistent set of co-morbidities that was reported in the studies we indentified, such that the significance of reported associations may be due, in part, to publication bias; the co-morbidities most strongly associated with events might have been more likely to have been reported. The following factors were all associated with bleeding in at least one of the studies: diabetes, kidney impairment, alcohol abuse, history of GI bleeds, prior stroke, hypertension, psychiatric illness, liver disease, anemia, leukoaraiosis (an age-related change in cerebral white matter), congestive heart failure, cancer, and venous thrombosis. Estimating the actual magnitude of each of these conditions' associations with serious bleeding is beyond the scope of this project and would be difficult given the available data. Particularly important to the task of estimating the impact of these conditions would be untangling the intensity of warfarin therapy and other potential confounding factors that might be mediating the associations with serious bleeding events.

Risk Indices

Several bleeding risk indices are currently available for stratifying patients into "low" and "high" risk groups. We identified seven articles[51,56,66,68,69,78,80] that estimated the risk of serious bleeding events in people on warfarin therapy using one or more of nine different risk indices (OBRI,[51] Shireman,[66] Kuijier,[83] AFI, ACCP, CHADS$_2$,[84] HEMORR2HAGES,[80] Kearon, NICE). Typically, these risk indices place patients into low, intermediate and high risk groups using several risk factors. Four of the risk indices (AFI, ACCP, CHADS$_2$, NICE)[78] were developed to predict risk of stroke, but also provided some evidence about whether or not they also predicted risk of serious bleeding complications. The stroke risk models appeared to be inferior to the bleeding risk models and likely only provide value for risk stratifying in studies that only have the stroke risk indices measured. Therefore, while the results from the stroke models are included in Appendix

B, Table 5, we will focus on the indices developed specifically for bleeding risk.

All of the risk indices included a categorical indicator of age as a component, but they differed in the age cut point with the age ≥60 used by the Kuijers risk index while others used ≥65, ≥70, ≥75, or a two level indicator with some increased risk at ≥65 and more risk ≥75. All of the indices included some increased risk for comorbidities. The comorbidities varied, particularly between the models that were designed specifically to predict stroke versus those designed to predict bleeding. The bleeding models tended to include some marker of prior history of bleeding events while the stroke models focused more on hypertension, history of stroke or TIA, or other vascular diseases. Most included diabetes mellitus as a risk factor and two of three bleeding models included female gender as a risk factor.[66,83]

Risk indices are difficult to compare across different studies. Two articles did however show head-to-head comparisons of different bleeding risk indices within the same study.[66,80] All of the bleeding risk indices were able to separate out groups of people with lower average risks of bleeding from those with higher risks of bleeding. Those identified as low risk typically have a several-fold lower risk of bleeding events compared to those identified as high risk. The amount of separation depended in part on the population. For example, a population where most of the patients are generally at a low risk of major bleeding will tend to show little separation, because there is not much of a range in risk. Likewise if age is an important factor in risk stratifying patients, using a tool with an age cut-off at age 65 for the higher risk group will not be very useful in a population where most of the patients are in their 70s or 80s.

Overall, while there have not been a lot of confirmatory studies of individual risk indices, bleeding risk indices were generally successful to some extent in stratifying patients into different risk groups. The choice of risk index might depend in part on the overall risk profile of the patient population (i.e., if many are well over age 65 then indices with older age cut-points might be more useful) and the availability of risk factor information (i.e., information on genotype status and level of detail on prior medical history).

SUMMARY – KEY QUESTION 3

Several individual risk factors (including very old age, initial warfarin use, INR variability, concomitant medications, comorbid conditions, mechanical heart valve, genetics) and combinations of risk factors (risk indices) can be used to define low and high risk groups for serious bleeding with warfarin use. However, due to the heterogeneity of studies (populations, risk factors assessed, risk factor definitions, etc.), it is difficult to reach definitive conclusions about the value of risk factor assessment.

Table 12. Risk Factors for Serious Bleeding Reported in the Individual Studies

Article	Age	Gender	Warfarin Duration	INR	Primary Indication	Asprin/ NSAID	Other Meds	Risk Index	Genetics	Co-morbidity	Other
Aspinall 2005[56]								✓			
Battistella 2005[57]										✓	
Beyth 1998[51]	✓		✓			✓	✓	✓			
Bousser 2008[66]											
DiMarco 2005[58]	✓					✓	✓	✓		✓	
Douketis 2006[62]	✓		✓			✓	✓			✓	
Douketis 2007[67]						✓	✓				
Fang 2005[59]		✓									
Fang 2006[64]	✓		✓								
Fihn 1996[49]	✓										
Flaker 2006[63]						✓					
Gage 2006[80]						✓	✓	✓			
Gasse 2005[60]											
Gomberg-M 2006[65]	✓	✓									
Hart 1999[53]						✓					
Healey 2008[69]								✓			
Higashi 2002[54]									✓		
Johnson 2008[70]						✓	✓			✓	
Le Tourneau 2009[81]				✓							
Limdi 2008[71]									✓	✓	
Limdi 2009[75]											
Lind 2009[77]	✓	✓									✓
Lindh 2008[72]	✓	✓	✓				✓				✓
McMahan 1998[52]	✓	✓				✓	✓			✓	✓
Meckley 2008[73]									✓		
Metlay 2008[74]			✓		✓	✓	✓				✓
Poli 2009b[78]	✓							✓			
Poli 2009a[76]	✓										
Schauer 2005[61]	✓	✓								✓	✓
Schelleman 2010[79]	✓									✓	
Shireman 2006[66]	✓	✓					✓	✓		✓	✓
Smith 2002[55]										✓	
SPAF 1996[48]	✓	✓				✓	✓			✓	✓
Van Leeuwen 2008[82]				✓							
White 1996[50]	✓	✓			✓					✓	✓
TOTAL (35)	16	9	5	2	2	11	11	7	3	12	8

DISCUSSION AND RECOMMENDATIONS

KEY QUESTION 1

For management of long-term outpatient anticoagulation in adults, are specialized anticoagulation clinics (ACC) more effective and safer than care in non-specialized clinics (e.g., primary care clinics, physician offices)?

Major Clinical Outcomes

The literature available to address this question is limited. We were able to identify 11 studies, of which only 3 were RCTs.[6,7,8] Except for one study,[14] major clinical outcomes occurred more frequently in the control than the intervention group (Table 3b). However, pooled results from the 3 RCTS showed no significant differences between ACC and UC for deaths, thromboembolic events, or major bleeding. Pooling of the observational studies' results was not possible due to heterogeneity among studies in reported outcome metrics.

Time in Therapeutic Range

All 9 studies that reported this metric (or the related metric, % INRs within therapeutic range) found that subjects receiving care in an ACC spent more time within the therapeutic range than those who received usual care.[6-8,10-14,16] In 4 studies the difference was statistically significant.[7,10,12,14] In the RCTs, the pooled weighted means were only slightly higher for ACC than UC (59.9% v.56.3%). In the observational studies, there was a larger spread with ACC patients spending 63.5% of the time in therapeutic range compared to 53.5% for subjects in usual care.

Patient Satisfaction

Measured in 2 of the RCTs, patient satisfaction was found to be significantly higher in patients randomized to the ACC intervention than to UC.[6,7]

Other Reviews

The 2008 ACCP guidelines on *Pharmacology and Management of the Vitamin K Antagonists*[1] included a narrative review of 9 uncontrolled studies, 3 cohort studies, and 2 RCTs. The authors concluded that *"although the literature … is not as robust as one would like, and there is great heterogeneity between studies, the results are almost always consistent, indicating that care provided by an anticoagulation management service results in better outcomes or more stable therapy than UC"* (p 184s[1]). Similarly a systematic review and meta-regression published in 2006[85] found that care provided in community settings resulted in significantly worse anticoagulation control (as measured by TTR) than that provided within ACCs (or within clinical trials). This review included studies of any design as long as the report included original data measuring serial INRs in at least one patient group. A third review and meta-analysis of 36 studies of patients with atrial fibrillation found that significantly more time was spent within the therapeutic range when patients were cared for in organized settings (i.e., ACCs) as compared with usual care.[86] Finally, a very recent meta-analysis investigated the effect of study-level factors (e.g., study design, year of publication, INR interpolation method) on time in therapeutic range and reported that patients managed in ACCs spent significantly more time within the therapeutic range than those managed in usual care.[87] None of these reviews evaluated clinical outcomes.

KEY QUESTION 1A

Which components of a specialized anticoagulation clinic are associated with effectiveness/ safety?

None of the included studies reported the association between specific elements of ACC and outcomes. Some possible processes of care that might have accounted for observed differences in outcomes in these studies included use of both face-to face and telephone interactions with patients;[13] use of a computerized patient monitoring system that identified patients who were delinquent in returning for timely INR determinations;[12] the specialized expertise of the ACC staff;[12] more consistency in ACCs in obtaining regular INRs;[11] and frequency of face-to-face consultations, methods of dosage adjustment, and provision of written dosage instructions.[16]

CONCLUSION AND RECOMMENDATIONS FOR KQ1

The evidence suggests that care provided within ACCs *may* lead to better quality anticoagulation control as measured by time in therapeutic range (a surrogate outcome that has been correlated with clinical events),[50] but there is insufficient evidence to conclude that ACC care leads to fewer deaths, thromboembolic events, or major bleeding events than care provided in usual care settings such as primary care clinics. Patients reported that they liked the convenience and enhanced service provided by ACCs. There is insufficient evidence for the VA to actively promote the implementation of ACCs. Other organizations have suggested greater benefits with ACCs; future research should include cost and resource utilization outcomes along with clinical outcomes and patient satisfaction measures. Future research should also address whether the benefits from ACC are restricted to the initiation of anticoagulation (a high risk period) or also continue through the maintenance phase.

KEY QUESTION 2

Is Patient Self Testing (PST), either alone or in combination with Patient Self Management (PSM), more effective and safer than standard care delivered in either ACCs or non-specialized clinics?

This analysis of 22 randomized, controlled trials (RCTs) indicates that for selected patients, oral anticoagulation therapy delivered through a PST/PSM model results in superior patient outcomes compared with oral anticoagulation therapy delivered through usual clinic based models. Patients randomized to PST/PSM, had a significant 26% lower risk of death and a significant 42% reduction in major thromboembolism without any increased risk of major bleeding events. We included between 4-12 more trials and 3500-5000 more patients than other meta-analyses[2,46,47,88] and to our knowledge we are the first to include the largest trial to date, *The Home INR Study*, a VA cooperative studies trial[17].

The mechanism by which PST/PSM leads to a reduction in thromboembolic events is thought to involve the higher proportion of time spent within the therapeutic range that is achieved with more frequent monitoring and dosage adjustments. This assumption has been predicated on observational data suggesting that the incidence of bleeding and thromboembolism is correlated with the quality of anticoagulation control (i.e., time in therapeutic range or % INR values within therapeutic range).[89-93] The recent VA trial also found a modest but statistically significant higher percent time within therapeutic range for patients randomized to PST than to usual care (absolute difference 3.8 percentage points).[17] Our study did not confirm this association, possibly because our analysis, which included the largest number of trials to-date, was limited to RCTs whereas other reports were either from single RCTs,[17,91,94] reviews that included both RCTS and observational studies,[89] database analyses[90,92] or retrospective cohort studies.[93]

It is important to note that these trials enrolled highly selected populations. Subjects had to have the desire and confidence as well as the manual dexterity, visual acuity, and mental faculties to use the testing device and either relay those values to their clinic (PST) or perform dose adjustment on their own (PSM). In most of the trials, 50% or fewer patients met preliminary eligibility criteria, successfully completed the training, and agreed to be randomized. Some of the reasons cited for patient unwillingness to participate or continue with the PST/PSM included patient-perceived physical limitations, lack of confidence in their ability to follow the protocol, difficulty performing measurements, and preference for an alternative method.[25,46] However, among the randomized patients, the percentage who continued with the intervention throughout the study was relatively high (64-98%) and patients in the PST/PSM group generally reported higher satisfaction and quality of life than those in usual care.

Several limitations of this analysis should be acknowledged. First, the methodological quality of the included trials was variable; only 5 trials met all of our quality indicators. Second, it is unclear whether the apparent benefits of PST/PSM result from the PST/PSM or simply from the more intense education that these patients receive. Third, the current data do not address the question of whether PST/PSM is safe during the high-risk initiation phase or should only be implemented during the maintenance phase. However, it is reassuring to note that in the VA trial there was no outcome difference between the group who had been randomized within 3 months of starting anticoagulation and the group that had been anticoagulated for more than 3 months.[17] Finally, the data on quality of life and patient satisfaction is difficult to interpret due to the wide range and variable quality of the outcome measures used.

Whether the results of this review can be applied to US health care systems is unclear. Only 2 of the 22 reviewed trials were conducted in the US[17,18] and both investigated PST not PSM. Furthermore, one of these, the VA trial, did not show a significant benefit among patients randomized to PST compared to those randomized to a high quality ACC. The generalizability of results from non-US trials to US health care settings is problematic since half of these trials used vitamin K antagonists not widely used in the US and several of these have markedly different half lives from warfarin.[1] Also, since PST/PSM is a complex multi-component intervention, it is important to have evidence of effectiveness in typical US healthcare settings. Finally, although we did not examine costs, survey data suggest that costs are likely to be a barrier to implementation.[95] Several cost analyses have concluded that implementing PST/PSM may not be cost-effective due to the high cost of the portable monitoring devices and supplies and of patient training.[2,96]

CONCLUSION AND RECOMMENDATIONS FOR KQ2

This analysis indicates that compared to usual clinic care, patient self testing with or without self management is associated with significantly fewer deaths and thromboembolic events without any increase in bleeding complications, for a select group of motivated patients requiring long term anticoagulation with Vitamin K antagonists. It should be noted, however, that while the strength of evidence was moderate for the thromboembolism and bleeding, it was low for mortality. Whether this care model is cost-effective and can be implemented successfully in typical US health care settings requires further study.

KEY QUESTION 3

What are the risk factors for serious bleeding in patients on chronic anticoagulant therapy?

Summary

Many factors have been shown to predict an increased risk of serious bleeding; however, there is no standard set of variables that is commonly reported such that coming up with a comprehensive list of independent risk factors is difficult and involves piecing together results from a very heterogeneous group of studies. Factors that seemed most consistently associated with serious bleeding included: very old age, the first months following warfarin initiation, other medication use (particularly aspirin use), comorbid conditions (such as history of GI bleeding events or diabetes), primary indication for taking warfarin was a valve condition, and genetic factors (ex. variation in the CYP2C gene). There have also been a number of studies of indices that pool together several of the before mentioned risk factors and shown that patients can to some extent be categorized into low, intermediate, and higher risk for serious bleeding events. Those identified as low risk typically have a several-fold lower risk of bleeding events compared to those identified as high risk. The amount of separation depended in part on the population. For example a population where most of the patients are generally at a low risk of major bleeding will tend to show little separation, because there is not much of a range in risk.

Limitations

Publication bias and the inability to pool results across studies due the heterogeneity of the study designs, analytical methods, and risk factors assessed limit the certainty that can be assigned to the results presented in this section. Publication bias is a concern when looking at lists of predictors of outcomes from observational studies. It is not uncommon for studies to evaluate associations for many more factors than they report results, creating a situation where, positive associations with bleeding may be more often reported than null associations. This may make some factors look artificially more strongly associated than they might be expected to be in real-world circumstances. For this reason, it is important to confirm more novel associations in large prospective studies. The range of uncertainty around the magnitude of effect for any of these risk factors is also necessarily large, since the heterogeneity of the studies precludes anything but a narrative review of the findings.

CONCLUSION AND RECOMMENDATIONS FOR KQ3

Several factors have been shown to consistently predict an increased risk of bleeding and, when pooled together, a subset of these risk factors has been shown to stratify groups of patients into lower and higher risk groups. Either alone or in combination, these risk factors can likely be used to help clinicians and patients have a dialog about the risks of warfarin therapy. Currently, there is not adequate evidence to suggest that any of the bleeding risk indices are meaningfully superior to the other indices. The HEMORR$_2$HAGES index seems to be the most comprehensive list of potential factors, while the OBRI index has been the most frequently tested model and is more parsimonious. While neither of these is clearly superior, it does seem that there is growing support for the development of more formal methods of risk assessment beyond that of simple clinical intuition or judgment, and the current risk indices provide a means to begin to be develop useful clinical support tools that can be tweaked as new risk factors are identified.

Future studies might better define the utility of these risk indices by randomizing patients to different bleed risk management strategies possibly incorporating different combinations of risk factors or bleeding risk indices to assess the potential benefits and harms of different anti-coagulation strategies.

FUTURE DIRECTIONS

The questions addressed in this review may become moot within the next several years. Very recent randomized controlled trials suggest that direct thrombin inhibitors, drugs currently being evaluated for the United States market, and which do not require intensive monitoring, may be as safe and efficacious as vitamin K antagonists. Specifically, in large randomized trials, dabigatran has been shown to be equivalent to warfarin for the prevention of thromboembolic events in patients with chronic atrial fibrillation[97] and deep vein thrombosis.[98] The long term safety of these new agents is not yet established. In one trial,[97] myocardial infarction was more common among patients randomized to dabigatran than to warfarin, although this association was only marginally significant. Furthermore, liver function abnormalities were observed with use of an older direct thrombin inhibitor, ximelagatran,[98] although to date this has not been observed with dabigatran. Final FDA approval of these products may significantly alter the standard for anticoagulation therapy and subsequent monitoring.

REFERENCES

1. Ansell J, Hirsh J, Hylek E, et al. Pharmacology and management of the vitamin K antagonists: American College of Chest Physicians Evidence-Based Clinical Practice Guidelines (8th Edition). Chest 2008;133(6 Suppl):160S-98S.

2. Connock M, Stevens C, Fry-Smith A, et al. Clinical effectiveness and cost-effectiveness of different models of managing long-term oral anticoagulation therapy: a systematic review and economic modelling. Health Technology Assessment (Winchester, England) 2007; 11(38):iii-iv.

3. Review Manager (RevMan) [Computer program]. Version 5.0 for Windows. Copenhagen: The Nordic Cochrane Centre, The Cochrane Collaboration, 2008.

4. Higgins JP, Thompson SG, Deeks JJ, Altman DG. Measuring inconsistency in meta-analysis. BMJ 2003;327:557-60.

5. Egger M, Davey Smith G, Schneider M, Minder C. Bias in meta-analysis detected by a simple, graphical test. BMJ 1997;315:629-34.

6. Wilson SJ, Wells PS, Kovacs MJ, et al. Comparing the quality of oral anticoagulant management by anticoagulation clinics and by family physicians: a randomized controlled trial. CMAJ 2003;169(4):293-8.

7. Chan FW, Wong RS, Lau WH, et al. Management of Chinese patients on warfarin therapy in two models of anticoagulation service - a prospective randomized trial. Br J Clin Pharmacol 2006;62(5):601-9.

8. Matchar DB, Samsa GP, Cohen SJ, et al. Improving the quality of anticoagulation of patients with atrial fibrillation in managed care organizations: results of the managing anticoagulation services trial. Am J Med 2002;113(1):42-51.

9. Lee YP, Schommer JC, Lee YP, et al. Effect of a pharmacist-managed anticoagulation clinic on warfarin-related hospital readmissions. Am JHealth-Syst Pharm 1996;53(13):1580-3.

10. Chiquette E, Amato MG, Bussey HI, et al. Comparison of an anticoagulation clinic with usual medical care: anticoagulation control, patient outcomes, and health care costs. Arch Intern Med 1998;158(15):1641-7.

11. Chamberlain MA, Sageser NA, Ruiz D, et al. Comparison of anticoagulation clinic patient outcomes with outcomes from traditional care in a family medicine clinic. J Am Board Fam Pract 2001;14(1):16-21.

12. Witt DM, Sadler MA, Shanahan RL, et al. Effect of a centralized clinical pharmacy anticoagulation service on the outcomes of anticoagulation therapy. Chest 2005;127(5):1515-22.

13. Nichol MB, Knight TK, Dow T, et al. Quality of anticoagulation monitoring in nonvalvular atrial fibrillation patients: comparison of anticoagulation clinic versus usual care. Ann Pharmacother 2008;42(1):62-70.

14.   Du X, Ma CS, Liu XH, et al. Anticoagulation control in atrial fibrillation patients present to outpatient clinic of cardiology versus anticoagulant clinics. Chin Medl J 200520;118(14):1206-9.

15.   Wallvik J, Sjalander A, Johansson L, et al. Bleeding complications during warfarin treatment in primary healthcare centres compared with anticoagulation clinics. Scand J Prim Health Care 2007;25(2):123-8.

16.   Ansell J, Hollowell J, Pengo V, et al. Descriptive analysis of the process and quality of oral anticoagulation management in real-life practice in patients with chronic non-valvular atrial fibrillation: the international study of anticoagulation management (ISAM). J Thromb Thrombolysis 2007;23(2):83-91.

17.   Matchar DM, Jacobson A, Dolor R, et al. for the THINRS Executive Committee and Site Investigators. Effect of home testing of international normalized ratio on clinical events. N Engl J Med 2010;363(17):1608-1620.

18.   Beyth RJ, Quinn L, Landefeld CS. A multicomponent intervention to prevent major bleeding complications in older patients receiving warfarin. A randomized, controlled trial. Ann Intern Med 2000;133(9):687-95.

19.   Sunderji R, Gin K, Shalansky K, et al. A randomized trial of patient self-managed versus physician-managed oral anticoagulation. Can J Cardiol 2004;20(11):1117-23.

20.   Sawicki PT. A structured teaching and self-management program for patients receiving oral anticoagulation: a randomized controlled trial. Working Group for the Study of Patient Self-Management of Oral Anticoagulation. JAMA 1999;281(2):145-50.

21.   Cromheecke ME, Levi M, Colly LP, et al. Oral anticoagulation self-management and management by a specialist anticoagulation clinic: a randomised cross-over comparison. Lancet 2000;356(9224):97-102.

22.   Fitzmaurice DA, Murray ET, Gee KM, et al. A randomised controlled trial of patient self management of oral anticoagulation treatment compared with primary care management. J Clin Pathol 2002;55(11):845-9.

23.   Gadisseur AP, Breukink-Engbers WG, van der Meer FJ, et al. Comparison of the quality of oral anticoagulant therapy through patient self-management and management by specialized anticoagulation clinics in the Netherlands: a randomized clinical trial. Arch Intern Med 2003;163(21):2639-46.

24.   Gadisseur AP, Kaptein AA, Breukink-Engbers WG, et al. Patient self-management of oral anticoagulant care vs. management by specialized anticoagulation clinics: positive effects on quality of life. J Thromb Haemost 2004;2(4):584-91.

25.   Khan TI, Kamali F, Kesteven P, et al. The value of education and self-monitoring in the management of warfarin therapy in older patients with unstable control of anticoagulation. Br J Haematol 2004;126(4):557-64.

26.   Gardiner C, Williams K, Mackie IJ, et al. Patient self-testing is a reliable and acceptable alternative to laboratory INR monitoring. Br J Haematol 2005;128(2):242-7.

27.   Voller H, Glatz J, Taborski U, et al. Self-management of oral anticoagulation in nonvalvular atrial fibrillation (SMAAF study). Zeitschrift fur Kardiologie 2005;94(3):182-6.

28.   Christensen TD, Maegaard M, Sorensen HT, et al. Self-management versus conventional management of oral anticoagulant therapy: A randomized, controlled trial. Eur J Intern Med 2006;17(4):260-6.

29.   Christensen TD, Maegaard M, Sorensen HT, et al. Self- versus conventional management of oral anticoagulant therapy: effects on INR variability and coumarin dose in a randomized controlled trial. Am J Cardiovasc Drugs 2007;7(3):191-7.

30.   Gardiner C, Williams K, Longair I, et al. A randomised control trial of patient self-management of oral anticoagulation compared with patient self-testing. Br J Haematol 2006;132(5):598-603.

31.   Dauphin C, Legault B, Jaffeux P, et al. Comparison of INR stability between self-monitoring and standard laboratory method: preliminary results of a prospective study in 67 mechanical heart valve patients. Arch Cardiovasc Dis 2008;101(11-12):753-61.

32.   Ryan F, Byrne S, O'Shea S. Randomized controlled trial of supervised patient self-testing of warfarin therapy using an internet-based expert system. J Thromb Haemost 2009;7:1284-90.

33.   Horstkotte D, Piper C, Wiemer M, et al. Improvement of prognosis by home prothrombin estimation in patients with life-long anticoagulation therapy (Abstract). Eur Heart J 1996;17(Suppl):230.

34.   Horstkotte D, Piper C, Wiemer M. Optimal Frequency of Patient Monitoring and Intensity of Oral Anticoagulation Therapy in Valvular Heart Disease. J Thromb Thrombolysis 1998;5 Suppl 1(3):19-24.

35.   Koertke H, Minami K, Breymann T, et al. INR Self-management after mechanical heart faclve replacement: ESCAT (Early Self-Controlled Anticoagulation Trial). Z Cardiol 2001;90(Suppl 6);V1/118-124.

36.   Koertke H, Korfer R. International normalized ratio self-management after mechanical heart valve replacement: is an early start advantageous? Ann Thorac Surg 2001;72(1):44-8.

37.   Koertke H, Zittermann A, Wagner O, et al. Self-management of oral anticoagulation therapy improves long-term survival in patients with mechanical heart valve replacement. AnnThorac Surg 2007;83(1):24-9.

38.   Sidhu P, O'Kane HO. Self-managed anticoagulation: results from a two-year prospective randomized trial with heart valve patients. Ann Thorac Surg 2001;72(5):1523-7.

39.   Fitzmaurice DA, Murray ET, McCahon D, et al. Self management of oral anticoagulation: randomised trial. BMJ 2005;331(7524):1057.

40.   Jowett S, Bryan S, Murray E, et al. Patient self-management of anticoagulation therapy: a trial-based cost-effectiveness analysis. Br J Haematol 2006;134(6):632-9.

41.   Menendez-Jandula B, Souto JC, Oliver A, et al. Comparing self-management of oral anticoagulant therapy with clinic management: a randomized trial. Ann Intern Med 2005;142(1):1-10.

42.   Siebenhofer A, Rakovac I, Kleespies C, et al. Self-management of oral anticoagulation in the elderly: rationale, design, baselines and oral anticoagulation control after one year of follow-up. A randomized controlled trial. Thromb Haemost 2007;97(3):408-16.

43.   Siebenhofer A, Rakovac I, Kleespies C, et al. Self-management of oral anticoagulation reduces major outcomes in the elderly. A randomized controlled trial. Thromb Haemost 2008;100(6):1089-98.

44.   Eitz T, Schenk S, Fritzsche D, et al. International normalized ratio self-management lowers the risk of thromboembolic events after prosthetic heart valve replacement. Ann Thorac Surg 2008;85(3):949-54.

45.   Soliman Hamad MA, van Eekelen E, van Agt T, van Straten AHM. Self-management program improves antiocoagulation control and quality of life: a prospective randomized study. Eur J Cardiothroac Surg 2009;35:265-9.

46.   Heneghan C, Alonso-Coello P, Garcia-Alamino JM, Perera R, Meats E, Glasziou P. Self-monitoring of oral anticoagulation: a systematic review and meta-analysis. Lancet 2006;367:404-11.

47.   Garcia-Alamino JM, Ward AM, Alonso-Coello P, Perera R, Bankhead C, Fitzmaurice D, et al. Self-monitoring and self-management of oral anticoagulation. Cochrane Database of Systematic Reviews 2010;Issue 4. Art. No.: CD003839.

48.   Stroke Prevention in Atrial Fibrillation (SPAF) Investigators. Bleeding during antithrombotic therapy in patients with atrial fibrillation. Arch Intern Med 1996;156(4):409-16.

49.   Fihn SD, Callahan CM, Martin DC, et al. The risk for and severity of bleeding complications in elderly patients treated with warfarin. The National Consortium of Anticoagulation Clinics. Ann Intern Med 1996;124(11):970-9.

50.   White RH, McKittrick T, Takakuwa J, et al. Management and prognosis of life-threatening bleeding during warfarin therapy. National Consortium of Anticoagulation Clinics. Arch Intern Med 1996;156(11):1197-201.

51   Beyth RJ, Quinn LM, Landefeld CS. Prospective evaluation of an index for predicting the risk of major bleeding in outpatients treated with warfarin. Am J Med 1998;105(2):91-9.

52.   McMahan DA, Smith DM, Carey MA, et al. Risk of major hemorrhage for outpatients treated with warfarin. J Gen Intern Med 1998;13(5):311-6.

53.   Hart RG, Benavente O, Pearce LA. Increased risk of intracranial hemorrhage when aspirin is combined with warfarin: A meta-analysis and hypothesis. Cerebrovasc Dis 1999;9(4):215-7.

54.   Higashi MK, Veenstra DL, Kondo LM, et al. Association between CYP2C9 genetic variants and anticoagulation-related outcomes during warfarin therapy. JAMA 2002;287(13):1690-8.

55.   Smith EE, Rosand J, Knudsen KA, et al. Leukoaraiosis is associated with warfarin-related hemorrhage following ischemic stroke. Neurology 2002;59(2):193-7.

56.   Aspinall SL, DeSanzo BE, Trilli LE, et al. Bleeding Risk Index in an anticoagulation clinic. Assessment by indication and implications for care. J Gen Intern Med 2005;20(11):1008-13.

57.   Battistella M, Mamdami MM, Juurlink DN, et al. Risk of upper gastrointestinal hemorrhage in warfarin users treated with nonselective NSAIDs or COX-2 inhibitors. Arch Intern Med 2005;165(2):189-92.

58.   DiMarco JP, Flaker G, Waldo AL, et al. Factors affecting bleeding risk during anticoagulant therapy in patients with atrial fibrillation: observations from the Atrial Fibrillation Follow-up Investigation of Rhythm Management (AFFIRM) study. Am Heart J 2005;149(4):650-6.

59.   Fang MC, Singer DE, Chang Y, et al. Gender differences in the risk of ischemic stroke and peripheral embolism in atrial fibrillation: the AnTicoagulation and Risk factors In Atrial fibrillation (ATRIA) study. Circulation 2005;112(12):1687-91.

60.   Gasse C, Hollowell J, Meier CR, et al. Drug interactions and risk of acute bleeding leading to hospitalisation or death in patients with chronic atrial fibrillation treated with warfarin. Thromb Haemost 2005;94(3):537-43.

61.   Schauer DP, Moomaw CJ, Wess M, et al. Psychosocial risk factors for adverse outcomes in patients with nonvalvular atrial fibrillation receiving warfarin. J Gen Intern Med 2005;20(12):1114-9.

62.   Douketis JD, Arneklev K, Goldhaber SZ, et al. Comparison of bleeding in patients with nonvalvular atrial fibrillation treated with ximelagatran or warfarin: assessment of incidence, case-fatality rate, time course and sites of bleeding, and risk factors for bleeding. Arch Intern Med 2006;166(8):853-9.

63.   Flaker GC, Gruber M, Connolly SJ, et al. Risks and benefits of combining aspirin with anticoagulant therapy in patients with atrial fibrillation: an exploratory analysis of stroke prevention using an oral thrombin inhibitor in atrial fibrillation (SPORTIF) trials. Am Heart J 2006;152(5):967-73.

64.   Fang MC, Go AS, Hylek EM, et al. Age and the risk of warfarin-associated hemorrhage: the anticoagulation and risk factors in atrial fibrillation study. J Am Geriatr Soc 2006;54(8):1231-6.

65.   Gomberg-Maitland M, Wenger NK, Feyzi J, et al. Anticoagulation in women with non-valvular atrial fibrillation in the stroke prevention using an oral thrombin inhibitor (SPORTIF) trials. Eur Heart J 2006;27(16):1947-53.

66.   Shireman TI, Mahnken JD, Howard PA, et al. Development of a contemporary bleeding risk model for elderly warfarin recipients. Chest 2006;130(5):1390-6.

67.   Douketis JD, Melo M, Bell CM, et al. Does statin therapy decrease the risk for bleeding in patients who are receiving warfarin? Am J Med 2007;120(4):369 e9- e14.

68.   Bousser MG, Bouthier J, Buller HR, et al. Comparison of idraparinux with vitamin K antagonists for prevention of thromboembolism in patients with atrial fibrillation: a randomised, open-label, non-inferiority trial. Lancet 2008;371(9609):315-21.

69.   Healey JS, Hart RG, Pogue J, et al. Risks and benefits of oral anticoagulation compared with clopidogrel plus aspirin in patients with atrial fibrillation according to stroke risk: the atrial fibrillation clopidogrel trial with irbesartan for prevention of vascular events (ACTIVE-W). Stroke 2008;39(5):1482-6.

70.   Johnson SG, Rogers K, Delate T, et al. Outcomes associated with combined antiplatelet and anticoagulant therapy. Chest 2008;133(4):948-54.

71.   Limdi NA, McGwin G, Goldstein JA, et al. Influence of CYP2C9 and VKORC1 1173C/T genotype on the risk of hemorrhagic complications in African-American and European-American patients on warfarin. Clin Pharmacol Ther 2008;83(2):312-21.

72.   Lindh JD, Holm L, Dahl ML, et al. Incidence and predictors of severe bleeding during warfarin treatment. J Thromb Thrombolysis 2008;25(2):151-9.

73.   Meckley LM, Wittkowsky AK, Rieder MJ, et al. An analysis of the relative effects of VKORC1 and CYP2C9 variants on anticoagulation related outcomes in warfarin-treated patients. Thromb Haemost 2008;100(2):229-39.

74.   Metlay JP, Hennessy S, Localio AR, et al. Patient reported receipt of medication instructions for warfarin is associated with reduced risk of serious bleeding events. J Gen Intern Med 2008;23(10):1589-94.

75.   Limdi NA, Beasley TM, Baird MF, et al. Kidney function influences warfarin responsiveness and hemorrhagic complications. J Am Soc Nephrol 2009;20(4):912-21.

76.   Poli D, Antonucci, Grifoni E, Abbate R, Gensini GF, Prisco D. Bleeding risk during oral anticoagulation in atrial fibrillation patients older than 80 years. J Am Coll Cardiol 2009a;54(11):999-1002.

77.   Lind M, Boman K, Johansson L, et al. Thrombomodulin as a marker for bleeding complications during warfarin treatment. Arch Intern Med 2009;169(13):1210-5.

78.   Poli D, Antonucci E, Grifoni E, et al. Stroke risk in atrial fibrillation patients on warfarin. Predictive ability of risk stratification schemes for primary and secondary prevention. Thromb Haemost 2009b;101(2):367-72.

79.   Schelleman H, Bilker WB, Brensinger CM, Wan F, Yang Y-X, Hennessy S. Fibrate/statin initiation in warfarin users and gastrointestinal bleeding risk. Am J Med 2010;123:151-7.

80.   Gage BF, Yan Y, Milligan PE, et al. Clinical classification schemes for predicting hemorrhage: results from the National Registry of Atrial Fibrillation (NRAF). Am Heart J 2006;151(3):713-9.

81.   Le Tourneau T, Lim V, Inamo J, et al. Achieved anticoagulation vs prosthesis selection for mitral mechanical valve replacement. A population based outcome study. Chest 2009;136:1503-13.

82.   Van Leeuwen Y, Rosendaal FR, Cannegieter SC. Prediction of hemorrhagic and thrombotic events in patients with mechanical heart valve prostheses treated with oral anticoagulants. J Thromb Haemost 2008;6:451-6.

83.   Kuijer PM, Hutten BA, Prins MH, et al. Prediction of the risk of bleeding during anticoagulant treatment for venous thromboembolism. Arch Intern Med 1999;159(5):457-60.

84.   Gage BF, Waterman AD, Shannon W, et al. Validation of clinical classification schemes for predicting stroke: results from the National Registry of Atrial Fibrillation. JAMA 2001;285(22):2864-70.

85.   van Walraven C, Jennings A, Oake N, et al. Effect of study setting on anticoagulation control: a systematic review and metaregression. Chest 2006;129(5):1155-66.

86.   Dolan G, Smith LA, Collins S, Plumb JM. Effect of setting, monitoring intensity and patient experience on anticoagulation control: a systematic review and meta-analysis of the literature. Curr Med Res Opin 2008;24(5):1459-1472.

87.   Cios DA, Baker WL, Sander SD, Phung OJ, Coleman CI. Evaluating the impact of study-level factors on warfarin control in U.S.-based primary studies: a meta-analysis. Am J Health Syst Pharm 2009;66(10):916-925.

88.   Christensen TD, Johnsen SP, Hjortdal VE, Hasenkam JM. Self-management of oral anticoagulant therapy: a systematic review and meta-analysis. Int J Cardiol 2007;118:54-61.

89.   Oake N, Jennings A, Forster AJ, Fergusson D, Doucette S, van Walraven C. Anticoagulation intensity and outcomes among patients prescribed oral anticoagulant therapy: a systematic review and meta-analysis. Can Med Assoc J 2008;179:235-44.

90.   vanWalraven C, Oake N, Wells PS, Forster AJ. Burden of potentially avoidable anticoagulant-associated hemorrhagic and thromboembolic events in the elderly. Chest 2007;131:1508-15.

91.   Connolly SJ, Pogue J, Eikelboom J, Flaker G, Commerford P, Franzosi MG. Benefit of oral anticoagulant over antiplatelet therapy in atrial fibrillation depends on the quality of international normalized ratio control achieved by centers and countries as measured by time in therapeutic range. Circulation 2008;118:2029-37.

92. Jones M, McEwan P, Morgan CL, Peters JR, Goodfellow J, Currie CJ. Evaluation of the pattern of treatment, level of anticoagulation control, and outcomes of treatment with warfarin in patients with non-valvar atrial fibrillation: A record linkage study in a large British population. Heart 2005;91:472-77.

93. Veeger NJ, Piersma-Wichers M, Tijssen JG, Hillege HL, van der Meer J. Individual time within target range in patients treated with Vitamin K antagonists: Main determinant of quality of anticoagulation and predictor of clinical outcome. A retrospective study of 2300 consecutive patients with venous thromboembolism. Br J Haematol 2005;128:513-9.

94. White HD, Gruber M, Feyzi J, Kaatz S, Tse H-F, Husted S, et al. Comparison of outcomes among patients randomized to warfarin therapy according to anticoagulant control. Arch Intern Med 2007;167:239-45.

95. Wittkowsky AK, Sekreta CM, Nutescu EA, Ansell J. Barriers to patient self-testing of prothrombin time: National survey of anticoagulation practitioners. Pharmacotherapy 2005;25:265-9.

96. Ansell J, Jacobson A, Levy J, et al. Guidelines for implementation of patient self-testing and patient self-management of oral anticoagulation. International consensus guidelines prepared by International Self-Monitoring Association for Oral Anticoagulation. Int J Cardiol 2005;99(1):37-45.

97. Connolly SJ, Ezekowitz MD, Yusuf S, et al. Dabigatran versus warfarin in patients with atrial fibrillation. N Engl J Med 2009;361(12):1139-51.

98. Schulman S, Kearon C, Kakkar AK, et al. Dabigatran versus Warfarin in the Treatment of Acute Venous Thromboembolism. N Engl J Med 2009;361(24):2342-52.

APPENDIX A: PEER REVIEW COMMENTS AND RESPONSES

Reviewer Comment	Author Response
Overall	
You exhaustively synthesize the literature related to the questions you sought to answer. This was extremely professional and the product is truly authoritative.	Thank you
Re: the repeated messages about how warfarin is due to be replaced at any moment 1. I'm not sure this really belongs in an ESP because this is not part of the evidence base you were synthesizing. 2. I suspect we will still be using warfarin, at least for some patients, for at least the next 10 years, if not more. No alternative agent has received FDA approval.	We have deleted many of the messages about potential alternatives to warfarin (see additional responses below).
The report is a comprehensive review of anticoagulation management in the outpatient setting.	Thank you
Objectives, Scope, and Methods Clearly Described	
Each of these areas is clearly described.	NR*
Yes	NR
Yes	NR
a. Yes. Overall, this is a very thoughtful, thorough, and well written report that provides a comprehensive summary of three decades of research on management of oral anticoagulation. b. Although the questions addressed by the review are clinically quite relevant, in certain respects, however, it forces the analysis to address the clinical circumstances in a somewhat unrealistic manner. The management of oral anticoagulation is simplistically divided into two phases: initiation and maintenance. As the authors of this review have found, the highest risk of complications is during this period [initiation]. Once stability is achieved, the maintenance is oriented toward minimizing variation in the INR related to intercurrent illness, administration of drugs, changes in diet, etc. Research suggests the inherent variability during this latter phase also predicts likelihood of complications. The analytic framework adopted in this review treats these phases as one continuous process. It is likely that interventions studies, i.e., AC clinics and PST, and the risk factors for complications might be different according to the phase studied. c. It does not appear that the confounding effects of computerized dosing programs, protocols, or nomograms were considered. My bias is that much of any beneficial effect of ACCs reflect the standard use of protocols. Can you ascertain if some of the "control" clinics related to Question #1 were using such tools?	Thank you. b. We have reviewed the studies cited in the report and have added information about initiation and maintenance phases in the Overview of Included Studies sections for KQ1 and KQ2. c. We have added information about possible processes of care that might have accounted for observed differences under KQ1a.

Bias	
I believe there is significant bias shown in support of the direct thrombin inhibitors class and specially dabigatran which is yet to be approved for release to the US market (*see pages iii, iv, and vi of the Executive Summary for example*); these statements are all speculative and biased and should not be included in an evidence based report. A more benign and accurate statement to be considered that could be used once in the Executive Summary: "New anticoagulants which may offer the same clinical efficacy and safety profile as warfarin with considerable less monitoring are currently being evaluated for the US market. Final FDA approval of these products may significantly alter the standard for anticoagulation therapy and subsequent monitoring".	Thank you for the suggested wording. We have added a statement to the "Background" section of the Executive Summary and the "Discussion and Recommendations" section of the full report. We have deleted all other statements about direct thrombin inhibitors.
No	NR
There is no evidence in the report to support the conclusions regarding direct thrombin inhibitors and specifically dabigatran (see pages iii, iv, vi, and 46). This drug has not been approved by the FDA for use in the US and the report does not draw on any FDA documents surrounding this drug. There have been several drugs that showed exceptional promise in pre-marketing trials that have either been withdrawn from the market or had their use severely limited due to problems found during post-marketing surveillance. Stating that direct thrombin inhibitors are "poised to become the preferred treatment for long term anticoagulation" shows bias towards this class of drugs that is not supported by evidence in the report. The statement on page 46 ("The long term safety of these new agents is not yet established") is not included in the executive summary. I would recommend removing references to direct thrombin inhibitors from the report. If it is included, I would recommend just stating this class of drugs is currently in clinical trials and the role in therapy has not been defined but may impact the usage of warfarin.	We have added a statement to the "Background" section of the Executive Summary and the "Discussion and Recommendations" section of the full report. We have deleted all other statements about direct thrombin inhibitors.
No	NR
Other Published or Unpublished Studies	
Not that I am aware of	NR
No	NR
None to my knowledge	NR

Comment	Response
It is not clear that all studies have been included specifically: 1. Fihn SD et al. Ann Intern Med 1993;118:511-520 (addresses several risk factors presented in Table 12 including variability in INR) 2. Van Leeuwen Y et al. Thromb Haemost 2008;6:451-460 (addresses variability in INR as a risk factor) 3. LeTourneau T. Chest 2009;136:1503-1513 (addressed variability in INR as a risk factor) There is evidence that variability in INR is important during the maintenance phase and should be acknowledged in the review.	Fihn 1993 was excluded, because it was outside of the search window (1996 or later). Information for both Van Leeuwen 2008 and LeTourneau 2009 has now been added to the KQ3 section.

Additional Comments

Comment	Response
Page 23, paragraph 2 - change THIINRS to THIINRS	NR
There are multiple statements diminishing the usefulness of this review with the assumption that direct thrombin inhibitors will replace warfarin for anticoagulation since they do not require intensive monitoring. It seems premature to make this assumption based on recently published RCTs. While these studies report the efficacy of the new drug in clinical trial populations, the effectiveness (or cost-effectiveness) of these therapies in non-clinical trial settings remains to be seen.	We have added a statement to the "Background" section of the Executive Summary and the "Discussion and Recommendations" section of the full report. We have deleted all other statements about direct thrombin inhibitors.
The THIINRS final analyses have been completed and the main study paper is planned for submission in February 2010. An inquiry on whether the unpublished results can be included in the tables and meta-analysis could be sent to the CSPCC in Palo Alto.	We have been in contact with the CSPCC and including unpublished data is not an option.

a. Although the literature synthesis showed insufficient evidence to conclude that ACC care leads to fewer deaths, thromboembolic events, or major bleeding events than usual care, several expert reviews have concluded that better quality anticoagulation control typically seen within an ACC can infer better outcomes. This is discussed in Philips and Ansell (2008) and the ACCP Guidelines (2008). This review does discuss other reviews (pg. 46) but this disparity is not discussed in the Executive Summary. b. Other organizations that have focused on quality and safety have supported AC clinics (Joint Commission Sentinel Event Alert Issue 41; AHRQ Report #43, Part III, Chpt. 9). c. For the conclusion on page iv that states "there is insufficient evidence for the VA to actively promote the implementation of ACCs" I would recommend stating further that this has not been the conclusion of other organizations or expand on how the conclusion of the systematic review differs from conclusions of other organizations and experts in the field. d. I would recommend adding that this synthesis of the literature did not consider the cost-effectiveness of ACCs or resource utilization and therefore the conclusion that there is insufficient evidence is based solely on evidence regarding clinical outcomes and does not factor in patient satisfaction, costs, and resource utilization. As the VA does manage a large portion of their patients within AC clinics HSR&D may want to consider a study that looks at AC clinic patient management within the VA system and include these factors.	a. We have chosen to present the results from our review in the Executive Summary leaving comparisons to other studies in the Discussion section. In agreement with the ACCP Guidelines, we have noted the limited nature of the evidence in the Executive Summary. b. We have reviewed these documents. The Joint Commission Alert is based on a few studies (not a comprehensive review). The AHRQ Report was completed in 2001 and therefore does not include many of the studies cited in our review. c. We are limited to reaching conclusions based on the evidence. d. Cost-effectiveness was outside the scope of the report as defined by the Key Questions. We searched for but were unable to identify evidence-based data on resource utilization. Patient satisfaction results are included in our review. We agree that a study that includes costs and resource utilization would be worthwhile and we have added a statement to that effect in the Conclusions and Recommendations for Key Question 1.
In a couple of places, the authors indicate that the review may be of limited value because of the imminent introduction of direct thrombin inhibitors. Although this may well be true, reports of demise of vit K antagonists have been prevalent for 3 decades. Although these drugs have a narrow therapeutic ratio, they have an efficacy in preventing stroke of nearly 75%, higher, perhaps, than almost any other drug in regular therapeutic use. Given the fact that the drug itself is relatively inexpensive, must typically be taken for many years, and has a long track record, it may not be dislodged all that soon.	We have added a statement to the "Background" section of the Executive Summary and the "Discussion and Recommendations" section of the full report. We have deleted all other statements about direct thrombin inhibitors.

*No Response Needed

APPENDIX B: EVIDENCE TABLES

Appendix B, Table 1 – Randomized Controlled Trials for Anticoagulation Clinic versus Usual Care (KQ1)

Study Publication Year Country of Origin Funding source	Indication for anticoagulation Entrance criteria Duration of follow-up Mean age % Male Inception Cohort/Time on OAC prior to enrollment	Intervention Group (n) Control Group (n) Total sample size (N)	Outcomes evaluated*	Study quality
Matchar, et al.[8] 2002 USA Agency for Healthcare Research and Quality, DuPont Pharmaceuticals Company	Atrial fibrillation Age ≥ 65, atrial fibrillation, enrolled in 1 of 6 managed care organizations Mean Age: 76+ 7 % Male: 49 A follow-up period of the 9 months immediately after the anticoagulation service had attained the minimum enrollment Inception: unclear	Intervention Cluster: referred to ACC:173, not referred to ACC: 190 Control Cluster: 317 N=680 *2 Practice clusters within each site were randomized to either access or no access to an ACC. The intervention clusters did not HAVE to refer pts to the ACC.*	iii. VTE iv. Bleeding vii. Time in Therapeutic Range	Allocation concealment: NA Blinding: NR Intention-to-treat: NR Dropouts reported: yes
Wilson, et al.[6] 2003 Canada Queen Elizabeth II Health Sciences Centre Research Foundation (Halifax, NS), Physicians' Services Incorporated Foundation (Ottawa, ON), London Health Sciences Centre Internal research Fund (London, ON)	Mixed indications All patients expected to be on warfarin ≥ 3mo Mean Age: 61+ 15 years % Male: 58 Follow-Up: 3 months Inception (< 1 month): 81%	Intervention: ACC: 112 Control: family physician:109 N = 221	i. All cause mortality ii. Event related mortality iii. VTE iv. Bleeding v. Patient Satisfaction vii. Time in Therapeutic Range	Allocation concealment: yes Blinding: clinical event adjudication committee blinded Intention-to-treat: yes Dropouts reported: yes

Chan, et al.[7] 2006 China Health Care and Promotion Fund (Hong Kong)	Mixed indications All patients, age ≥ 18, requiring ≥ 3mo of warfarin therapy Mean Age: 59 + 14 years % Male: 45 Follow-Up: max 2 years, average length cannot be determined Inception cohort: see page 602	Intervention: pharmacist-managed ACC: 69 Control: hematologist-managed ACC: 69 N = 138	i. All cause mortality iii. VTE iv. Bleeding v. Patient Satisfaction vii. Time in Therapeutic Range xi. Hospitalization xii. Outpatient Utilization xiii. ER Utilization	Allocation concealment: unclear Blinding: NR Intention-to-treat: no Dropouts reported: yes

* OUTCOMES

i. All cause mortality
ii. Event related mortality
iii. VTE (venous thromboembolic events)
iv. Bleeding
v. Patient Satisfaction
vi. Quality of Life
vii. Time in Therapeutic Range

viii. % of INRs in Therapeutic Range
ix. INR Variability
x. # of Total INR Values
xi. Hospitalization
xii. Outpatient Utilization
xiii. ER Utilization
xiv. Outpatient Laboratory Utilization
xv. Long-term Care Admission
　　(after related event)

Appendix B, Table 2 – Observational Studies for Anticoagulation Clinic versus Usual Care (KQ1)

Study Publication Year Country of Origin Funding Source	Study design Indication for anticoagulation Entrance criteria Duration of follow-up Mean age % Male % Inception/time on OAC prior to enrollment	Intervention Group (n) Control Group (n) Total sample size (N)	Outcomes evaluated*
Lee, et al.[9] 1996 USA	Prospective Cohort Mixed indications All patients discharged from hospital requiring long term warfarin. Follow-Up: 3 mos Mean Age: 56.9 % Male: 57 Inception: NR	Intervention: Hospital discharges requiring long term anticoagulation referred to anticoagulation clinic. The ACC was led by a pharmacist and included patient education via manuals, videos and compliance aids. (68) Control: Random sample of hospital discharges requiring long term warfarin but not referred to anticoagulation clinic (68) N = 136	xi. Hospitalization
Chiquette, et al.[10] 1998 USA	Retrospective Cohort Mixed Indications All patients, requiring ≥3mo of warfarin therapy, with at least one outpatient visit Follow-Up: NR Mean Age: NR (90% < 65) % Male: 53 Inception: 100%	Intervention: ACC which was led by a pharmacist and included intensive patient education; no dosing algorithm (183) Control: Usual medical care (145) N = 328	iii. VTE iv. Bleeding vii. Time in Therapeutic Range viii. % of INRs in Therapeutic Range xi. Hospitalization xiii. ER Utilization
Chamberlain, et al.[11] 2001 USA Southwest Washington Medical Center	Retrospective Cohort Mixed indications All anticoagulation patients during study period included Follow-Up: NR Mean Age: 63 + 15 % Male: 42 Inception: No/NR	Intervention: Anticoagulation patients during the period 11/1/1996 to 10/31/1997 followed in a pharmacist-run anticoagulation clinic which included POC testing (41) Control: Anticoagulation patients during the period 11/1/1996 to 10/31/1997 followed in a family medicine clinic that did not perform POC testing (75) N = 116	iii. VTE viii. % of INRs in Therapeutic Range xi. Hospitalization xiii. ER Utilization
Witt, et al.[12] 2005 USA	Retrospective Cohort Mixed indications ≥ 18yo, on warfarin, ≥2 INR values during 6 mo evaluation period Follow-Up: 6 months Mean Age: 67.8 % Male: 53 Inception:NR	Intervention: Anticoagulation therapy managed by a centralized, telephonic clinical pharmacy anticoagulation service manned by pharmacists available 24/7; patient education provided (3323) Control: Anticoagulation therapy managed per usual personal physician. (3322) N = 6645	i. All cause mortality ii. Event related mortality iii. VTE iv. Bleeding vii. Time in Therapeutic Range

Safe and Effective Anticoagulation in the Outpatient Setting

Du, et al.[14] 2005 China	Prospective cohort Atrial fibrillation NVAF on anticoagulation Follow-Up: NR Mean Age: 61.8 % Male: 59 Inception: NR	Intervention: referred to anticoagulation clinic (details not provided) (66) Control: followed by usual care which consists of follow-up by cardiology outpatient clinic (138) N = 204	iii. VTE iv. Bleeding viii. % of INRs in Therapeutic Range
Ansell, et al.[16] 2007 USA, Sweden, Italy, Spain, France AstraZeneca Pharmaceuticals	Retrospective Cohort Atrial fibrillation Cross-sectional cohort with chronic NVAF, age >18, minimum 60 days of AC Follow-Up: 12 months Mean Age: NR % Male: NR Inception: NR	Intervention: Patients of anticoagulation clinics using local protocols were followed in Italy and Spain. ACC management was defined as care provided in a systematic way by personnel focusing specifically on AC management (395) Control: Patients of routine medical care using local protocols were followed in the US, Canada and France (1116) N = 1511	vii. Time in Therapeutic Range viii. % of INRs in Therapeutic Range
Wallvik, et al.[15] 2007 Sweden Joint Committee of Northern Sweden Health Care Region and Foundation of Medical Research in Skelleftea	Prospective Cohort Mixed indications All patients treated with warfarin in two regions of northern Sweden. Follow-Up: 1.8 years (mean), 4 yrs max Mean Age: 69 % Male: 58 Inception cohort: NR	Intervention: Anticoagulation clinic, no details provided (1537) Control: Primary healthcare centre (1194) N = 2731	iv. Bleeding
Nichol, et al.[13] 2008 USA AstraZeneca Pharmaceuticals	Retrospective Cohort Atrial Fibrillation NVAF on anticoagulation Follow-Up: 12 mos Mean Age: NR % Male: 55 Inception: No	Intervention: ACC run by an RN mostly by phone, supervised by a cardiologist; intensive pt education on first visit. (351) Control: Usual care by internists, GPs or cardiologists. (756) N = 1107	iii. VTE iv. Bleeding vii. Time in Therapeutic Range

*OUTCOMES

i. All cause mortality
ii. Event related mortality
iii. VTE (venous thromboembolic events)
iv. Bleeding
v. Patient Satisfaction
vi. Quality of Life

vii. Time in Therapeutic Range
viii. % of INRs in Therapeutic Range
ix. INR Variability
x. # of Total INR Values
xi. Hospitalization
xii. Outpatient Utilization

xiii. ER Utilization
xiv. Outpatient Laboratory Utilization
xv. Long-term Care Admission (after related event)

Appendix B, Table 3 – Overview of individual short-term (<12 months) randomized, controlled trials investigating PST/PSM (KQ2)

Study Publication year Country of origin Funding source	Indications for anticoagulation Entrance criteria Duration of follow-up Mean age % Male Length of time on OAC prior to enrollment	Intervention group (n) Control group (n) Total sample size (N) Type of vitamin K antagonist	Outcomes evaluated*	Study quality
Sawicki et al. 1999[20] Germany Industry	Mixed Patients with a disease or condition requiring lifelong OAC 6 months 55±12 years 70% male 2.1±4.8 years (mean) Not clear (pts were not previously treated in THESE clinics)	Intervention: PSM (n=90) Control: PC clinic (n=89) N=179 Phenprocoumon	iii. Thromboembolic events iv. Major bleeding events v. Patient satisfaction/ quality of life vii. INR variability	Allocation concealment: adequate Blinding: lab techs doing the INRs were blinded Intention-to-treat: yes Dropouts reported: yes
Beyth et al. 2000[18] USA NIH, VA HSR&D, American Federation for Aging Research	Mixed Patients aged ≥65 years, residing in Cuyahoga County, OH, starting on OAC with treatment planned for ≥10 days 6 months 75 ± 6.8 years (range 65-94) 43% male 0 years (inception cohort)	Intervention: PST (n=163) Control: PC clinic (n=162) N=325 Warfarin	i. All-cause mortality iii. Thromboembolic events iv. Major bleeding events vii. % time within therapeutic range	Allocation concealment: unclear Blinding: two author-reviewers who were blinded to group assignment adjudicated bleeding events Intention-to-treat: yes Dropouts reported: yes
Cromheecke et al. 2000[21] Crossover trial The Netherlands Not reported	Mixed Self-supporting patients receiving long-term OAC 6 months (each pt followed 3 mos in each treatment) 42 ± 16 years (range 21-71) 59% male 3.9±2.2 years (mean) (not inception)	Intervention: PSM (n=50) Control: AC clinic (n=50) (Total N=50) Phenprocoumon and acenocoumarol	iii. Thromboembolic events iv. Major bleeding events v. Patient satisfaction/ quality of life vi. % time within therapeutic range vii. % INR values within therapeutic range	Allocation concealment: adequate Blinding: NR Intention-to-treat: unclear Dropouts reported: yes

Fitzmaurice et al. 2002[22] United Kingdom Industry	Mixed Patients aged ≥18 years, on long-term OAC for ≥6 months previously, with good vision and manual dexterity, and with INR within 0.5 of target value at least 60% of the time over the prior 12 months 6 months 66 years 76% male Not reported (not inception)	Intervention: PSM (n=30) Control: AC clinic (n=26) N=56 Warfarin	iv. Major bleeding events v. Patient satisfaction/ quality of life vi. % time within therapeutic range vii. % INR values within therapeutic range	Allocation concealment: unclear Blinding: no Intention-to-treat: no Dropouts reported: yes
Gadisseur et al. 2003[23] **& Gadisseur et al. 2004**[24] The Netherlands Industry	Mixed Patients aged 18-75, requiring long-term OAC, with ≥3 months experience on OAC 24.4 weeks (mean) 59 years 71% male Not reported (not inception)	Intervention (1): PST (n=52) Intervention (2): PSM (n=47) Control (1): AC clinic patients aware of the study and receiving education about OAC (n=60) Control (2): AC clinic patients not aware of the study (n=161) N=320 Phenprocoumon and acenocoumarol	iii. Thromboembolic events iv. Major bleeding events v. Patient satisfaction/ quality of life vi. % time within therapeutic range vii. % INR values within therapeutic range	Allocation concealment: adequate Blinding: physicians evaluating and correcting the proposed dosing schedules for group A and group B Intention-to-treat: yes Dropouts reported: yes
Khan et al. 2004[25] United Kingdom BUPA Foundation	Atrial Fibrillation Patients aged ≥65 years without dementia, on warfarin for ≥12 months, with a target INR of 2-3, with an INR standard deviation of ≥ 0.5 over prior 6 months 6 months Median age 73 yrs (range: 65-93) 58% male Not reported (not inception)	Intervention: PST (n=44) Control (1): ACC patients aware of the study and receiving education about OAC (n=41) Control (2): ACC patients not aware of the study (n=40) N=125 Warfarin	iii. Thromboembolic events iv. Major bleeding events v. Patient satisfaction/ quality of life vi. % time within therapeutic range	Allocation concealment: unclear Blinding: NR Intention-to-treat: no Dropouts reported: yes

Study	Population	Intervention/Control	Outcomes	Quality
Sunderji et al. 2004[19] Canada Industry and others	Mixed Patients age ≥ 18 years on warfarin for ≥ 1 month with target INR range 2-3 or 2.5-3.5, without mental incompetence or known hypercoagulable disorders 8 months 60 years 71% male 53.5% with ≥ 6 months OAC	Intervention: PSM (n=70) Control: PC clinic (n=70) N=140 Warfarin	iii. Thromboembolic events iv. Major bleeding events v. Pt Satisfaction vi. % time within therapeutic range vii. % INR values within therapeutic range	Allocation concealment: adequate Blinding: no Intention-to-treat: yes Dropouts reported: yes
Gardiner et al. 2005[26] United Kingdom Industry	Mixed Patients aged ≥18 years attending the anticoagulation clinic at University College London Hospital, on OAC for ≥8 months, with previous record of good compliance 6 months 58 years (range 26-83) (unclear if mean or median) 63% male Not reported (not inception)	Intervention: PST (n=44) Control: AC clinic (40) N=84 Warfarin	iv. Major bleeding events v. Pt Satisfaction vi. % time within therapeutic range	Allocation concealment: unclear Blinding: no Intention-to-treat: unclear Dropouts reported: yes
Voller et al. 2005[27] Germany Industry	Atrial fibrillation Patients on OAC for atrial fibrillation, without alcoholism or other addictions 39±6 mos 64 ± 9.3years 66% male Not reported	Intervention: PSM (n=101) Control: PC clinic (n=101) N=202 Not reported	iii. Thromboembolic events iv. Major bleeding events vi. % time within therapeutic range (# of days) vii. % INR values within therapeutic range	Allocation concealment: unclear Blinding: no Intention-to-treat: unclear Dropouts reported: unclear
Christensen et al. 2006[28] **& Christensen et al. 2007**[29] Denmark Danish Heart Foundation	Mixed Patients aged ≥18 years on OAC for ≥8 months 182 days (mean) 49 ± 13.7 years 67% male 5.5±4.3 years (mean) Not reported (not inception)	Intervention: PSM (n=50) Control: PC/AC clinic (n=50) N=100 Warfarin and phenprocoumon	i. All-cause mortality iii. Thromboembolic events iv. Major bleeding events vi. % time within therapeutic range viii. INR variability	Allocation concealment: no Blinding: no Intention-to-treat: no Dropouts reported: yes

Study	Population	Intervention/Control	Outcomes	Quality
Gardiner et al. 2006[30] United Kingdom Industry	Mixed. Patients aged ≥18 years on long-term OAC for ≥8 months, without history of poor compliance, intellectual impairment, or known drug or alcohol dependency. 6 months. 60 years (22-88). 61% male. Not reported (not inception)	Intervention: PSM (n=55) Control: PST (n=49) N=104 Warfarin	vi. % time within therapeutic range	Allocation concealment: unclear Blinding: no Intention-to-treat: unclear Dropouts reported: yes
Dauphin et al. 2008[31] France Industry	MHV replacement. Patients undergoing mechanical valve replacement at Clermont-Ferrand University Hospital. 47 ± 12 weeks (mean). 57 ± 9.7 years. 67% male. Not reported (recruited when undergoing valve replacement)	Intervention: PST (n=33) Control: AC clinic (n=34) N=67 Fluindione and acenocoumarol	i. All-cause mortality iii. Thromboembolic events iv. Major bleeding events vi. % time within therapeutic range vii. % INR values within therapeutic range viii. INR variability	Allocation concealment: unclear Blinding: no Intention-to-treat: unclear Dropouts reported: yes
Ryan et al. 2009[32] Crossover trial Ireland Industry and Health Research Board, Ireland	Mixed. Patients on OAC for ≥2 months with internet access. 6 months. 58.7 ± 14.3 years. 62% male. Not reported (not inception)	Intervention: PSM (n=132 completed both arms,72 initially) Control: AC clinic (n=132,60 initially) N=162 Warfarin	iii. Thromboembolic events iv. Major bleeding events vi. % time within therapeutic range	Allocation concealment: adequate (pharmacy-controlled) Blinding: no Intention-to-treat: no Dropouts reported: yes

*OUTCOMES
i. All cause mortality
ii. Event related mortality
iii. VTE (venous thromboembolic events)
iv. Bleeding
v. Patient Satisfaction
vi. Quality of Life
vii. Time in Therapeutic Range

viii. % of INRs in Therapeutic Range
ix. INR Variability
x. # of Total INR Values
xi. Hospitalization
xii. Outpatient Utilization
xiii. ER Utilization

Appendix B, Table 4 – Overview of individual long-term (≥12 months) randomized, controlled trials investigating PST/PSM (KQ2)

Study Publication year Country of origin Funding source	Indications for anticoagulation Entrance criteria Duration of follow-up Mean age % Male Inception cohort/ time on OAC prior to enrollment	Intervention (n) Control (n) Total sample size (N) Type of vitamin K antagonist	Outcomes evaluated[*]	Study quality
Horstkotte et al. 1998[34], 1996[33] (abstract) Germany Not reported	MHV replacement Entrance criteria not reported 17.7 months (mean) Not reported Not reported Not reported	Intervention: PSM (n=75) (dosing unclear) Control: PC clinic (n=75) N=150 Not reported	iii. Thromboembolic events iv. Major bleeding events vii. % INR measurements within therapeutic range	Allocation concealment: unclear Blinding: NR Intention-to-treat: unclear Dropouts reported: unclear
Koertke et al. 2001 (one in German in Z Kardiol[35] and one in Ann Thor Surg[36]) & Koertke et al. 2007[37] Germany Not reported	MHV replacement Patients undergoing MHV replacement from 2/1994-10/1997 at a German institution Initial f/u: 38 mos Long-term f/u: 9.3 +/- 2.8 years 63 years 66% male Inception Cohort	Intervention: PSM (n=579 in 2001; 488 in 2007) Control: PC clinic (n=576 in 2001; 442 in 2007) N (2001)=1155 N (2007)=930 Phenprocoumon	i. All-cause mortality(2007) ii. Event-related mortality (2007) iii. Thromboembolic events (2001) iv. Major bleeding events (2001) vii. % INR values within therapeutic range (2001)	Allocation concealment: unclear Blinding: NR Intention-to-treat: unclear Dropouts reported: yes
Sidhu et al. 2001[38] United Kingdom Industry	MHV replacement Patients who had undergone MHV replacement by the author and were ≤ 85 yo without visual difficulties 24 months 61 years (range: 26-85) 46% male Not reported	Intervention: PSM (n=51) Control: PC or AC clinic (n=49) N=100 Warfarin	i. All-cause mortality ii. Event-related mortality iii. Thromboembolic events iv. Major bleeding events vi. % time within therapeutic range	Allocation concealment: unclear Blinding: NR Intention-to-treat: unclear Dropouts reported: yes

Study	Population	Intervention/Control	Outcomes	Quality
Fitzmaurice et al. 2005[39] & Jowett et al. 2006[40] United Kingdom United Kingdom Medical Research Council	Mixed Patients aged ≥18 years on warfarin for ≥6 months with treatment indicated for ≥12 months, with a target INR of 2.5-3.5 12 months 65 years 65% male Not reported (not inception)	Intervention: PSM (n=337) Control: AC clinic (n=280) N=617 Warfarin	i. All-cause mortality ii. Event-related mortality iii. Thromboembolic events iv. Major bleeding events v. Patient satisfaction/quality of life vi. % time within therapeutic range	Allocation concealment: adequate Blinding: no Intention-to-treat: yes Dropouts reported: yes
Menendez-Jandula et al. 2005[41] Spain Industry	Mixed Patients aged ≥18 years on long-term OAC for ≥3 months, without severe physical or mental illness 12 months (median f/u) 65 years 53% male 5.1 years (median, IQR 2.0-12.0) % inception NR	Intervention: PSM (n=368) Control: AC clinic (n=369) N=737 acenocoumarol	i. All-cause mortality iii. Thromboembolic events iv. Major bleeding events vi. % time within therapeutic range vii. % INR values within therapeutic range viii. INR variability (INR distance, table 2)	Allocation concealment: adequate Blinding: complications diagnosed and evaluated by a third physician not involved in the trial and unaware of patients' study group Intention-to-treat: yes Dropouts reported: yes
Siebenhofer et al. 2007[42] & Siebenhofer et al. 2008[43] Austria Industry	Mixed Patients aged ≥60 years, on long-term OAC, without severe cognitive problems or terminal illness 2.9 ± 1.2 years (mean) 69 ± 6.3 years 58% male 5.7 ±7.1 years (mean) Not inception	Intervention: PSM (n=99) Control: AC/PC clinic (n=96) N=195 Phenprocoumon and acenocoumarol	i. All-cause mortality ii. Event-related mortality (see table 4 p. 1096) iii. Thromboembolic events iv. Major bleeding events vi. % time within therapeutic range vii % INR values within therapeutic range viii. INR variability	Allocation concealment: adequate Blinding: complications evaluated by two independent physicians not involved in the trial and unaware of patients' study group. Intention-to-treat: yes Dropouts reported: yes

Study	Population / Setting	Intervention / Control	Outcomes*	Quality
Eitz et al. 2008[44] Germany Not reported	MHV replacement Patients undergoing MHV replacement in a German hospital 2 years 58.7 years 69% male Not reported (randomized at time of valve replacement)	Intervention: PSM (n=470) Control: PC clinic (n=295) (crossovers were allowed) N=765 Warfarin	iii. Thromboembolic events iv. Major bleeding events vii. % INR values within therapeutic range viii. INR variability	Allocation concealment: unclear Blinding: NR Intention-to-treat: no Dropouts reported: no
Soliman Hamad 2009[45] The Netherlands Not reported	MHV replacement Patients undergoing MHV replacement in a Dutch hospital with knowledge of computers and the internet. 12 months 56 years Not reported Inception cohort (randomized at time of valve replacement)	Intervention: PSM (n=29) Control: AC clinic (n=29) N=62 Not reported	i. All-cause mortality iii. Thromboembolic events iv. Major bleeding events v. Pt Satisfaction /quality of life vi. % time within therapeutic range	Allocation concealment: unclear Blinding: NR Intention-to-treat: no Dropouts reported: yes
Matchar (THINRS) 2010[17] USA VA	Mixed Patients with MHV replacement or atrial fibrillation and competent in device use 2 to 4.75 years 67 ± 9 years 98% male Not an inception cohort (mean time on OAT prior to enrollment not reported)	Intervention: PST (n=1,465) Control: AC clinic (n=1,457) N=2922 Warfarin	i. All-cause mortality iii. Thromboembolic events iv. Major bleeding events v. Pt Satisfaction /quality of life vi. % time within therapeutic range	Allocation concealment: adequate Blinding: major outcomes assessed by independent adjudicators Intention-to-treat: yes Dropouts reported: yes

*OUTCOMES
i.   All cause mortality
ii. Event related mortality
iii. VTE (venous thromboembolic events)
iv. Bleeding
v.   Patient Satisfaction
vi. Quality of Life
vii. Time in Therapeutic Range
viii. % of INRs in Therapeutic Range
ix. INR Variability

x.   # of Total INR Values
xi. Hospitalization
xii. Outpatient Utilization
xiii. ER Utilization

Safe and Effective Anticoagulation in the Outpatient Setting

Appendix B, Table 5. Overview of Individual Studies – Risk Factors for Serious Bleeding (KQ3)

Study Country of origin Funding source	Study design Indications for anticoagulation Entrance criteria Duration of follow-up (years)	N (cases) Mean age % Male	Definition of Serious Bleeding	Serious Bleeding Outcomes by Risk Factors
Aspinall 2005[56] United States Public	Retrospective cohort study using Administrative Datasets. Patients attending a VA anticoagulation clinic between 2001 and 2002. Follow-up Administrative Data from January 1, 2001 to December 31, 2002	N(cases): 1,269 (42) Mean age: 67.9 (SD=11.4) 92% Male	Patient was hemo-dynamically unstable, required a transfusion, had an intracranial hemorrhage, or died.	*Risk Index* (Bleeding Risk Index) * Low: 0.8% /PYr (95% CI; 0-4.2) Med: 2.5%/PYr (95%CI;1.6-3.7) High: 10.6% /PYr (95% CI; 6.4-16.6) *Warfarin Duration* (p=.08)* New User (n/N): 2.2% (11/502) Prior User (n/N): 4.0% (31/767)
Battistella 2005[57] Canada Public	Nested case-control study using Administrative Datasets. Cohort of continuous warfarin users from April 1, 2000, to March 31, 2001. Follow-up 1 year	N(cases): 1,798 (361) Mean age: 77 (SD=6.8) 49% Male	Patient was admitted to the hospital with any diagnosis of upper GI hemorrhage	*Other Med Use**** NSAID: OR=1.9 (95%CI;1.4-3.7) Cox-2 Inhibitors Celecoxib: OR=1.7 (95%CI;1.2-3.6) Rofecoxib: OR=2.4 (95%CI;1.7-3.6)
Beyth 1998[51] United States Public	2 Prospective cohort studies (derivation and validation cohorts) using data primarily medical records. Derivation cohort of patients who started outpatient warfarin therapy upon discharge from hospital between 1977 and 1983. Validation inception cohort of consecutive patients who started warfarin therapy upon discharge from hospital between 1986 and 1987. Follow-up for both groups was presented up to 4 years.	**Derivation cohort:** N(cases): 565 (65) Mean age: 61(SD=14) 47% Male **Validation cohort:** N(cases): 264 (22) Mean age: 60(SD=16) 47% Male	Overt bleeding that led to the loss of at least 2.0 units in 7 days or less, or was otherwise life-threatening (eg. intracranial bleeding)	**Results from Derivation cohort:** *Risk Index (Outpatient Bleeding Risk Index)* Risk of major bleeding at 12 months Low: 3% Intermediate: 12% High: 48% *Warfarin Duration (follow-up time not time on warfarin)* Cumulative events at 1 month: 3% Cumulative events at 12 months: 11% Cumulative events at 48 months: 22% **Results from Validation cohort:** *Risk Index (Outpatient Bleeding Risk Index)* Risk of major bleeding at 12 months Low: 3% Intermediate: 8% High: 30% *Warfarin Duration (follow-up time not time on warfarin)* Cumulative events at 1 month: 2% Cumulative events at 12 months: 8 % Cumulative events at 48 months: 12% **Results from Combined Cohorts:** Stratifying by increased *Age* and *Comorbidity* (components of OBRI) shows increased the major bleeding

Safe and Effective Anticoagulation in the Outpatient Setting

Bousser 2008[68] Multi-national Industry	Prospective Cohort (vitamin K antagonist arm of RCT, warfarin or acenocoumarol) Patients with atrial fibrillation at risk for thromboembolism Follow-up 0.9 years (SD=0.5)	N(cases): 2293(29) Mean age: 70.2 (SD=9.1 65% Male	Bleeding that was fatal, intracranial, or affected another critical anatomical site, or overt bleeding with a drop of hemoglobin ≥20 g/L or requiring transfusion of two or more units of Erythrocytes.	**_Risk Index_** (CHADS2 score) * _Low:_ 0.8% /PYr _Moderate:_ 1.0% /PYr _High:_ 2.5% /PYr
DiMarco 2005[58] United States AFFIRM Trial Public	RCT comparing rate-control and rhythm-control strategies in patients with atrial fibrillation All patients were eligible for warfarin at baseline and most continued their warfarin regimen Follow-up average of 3.5 years (range 0 – 5.9 years)	N(cases): 4060 (260) Mean age: 70 (SD=9) 61% Male	Major bleeding was either CNS hemorrhage, or outside the CNS bleeding that required transfusion of ≥2 units of blood, hospitalization in an intensive care unit, and/or discontinuation of anticoagulant or antiplatelet Therapy.	**_Age:_** _(per year):_ HR=1.05(95%CI;1.04,1.07)*** **_Comorbidities:_** CHF: HR=1.43(95%CI;1.09,1.89)*** Diabetes: HR=1.44(95%CI;1.07,1.93)*** Hepatic or Renal Disease: HR=1.93(95%CI;1.27,2.93)*** **_Other Med Use:_** Aspirin Use: HR=2.01(95%CI;1.45,2.77)*** **_Rate Control vs. Rhythm-control strategies_** No difference (p=0.45)
Douketis 2006[62] Multinational SPORTIF III & V Trials Industry	Pooled analysis of two large RCTs using just the Warfarin arms of each trial Patients were adults with nonvalvular atrial fibrillation Followed up to 24 months	N(cases): 3665 (136) Mean age: ~71 <65: 22% 65-75: 40% >75: 38% 70% Male	Major bleeding was: fatal bleeding; clinically overt bleeding associated with a reduction in hemoglobin level of 20 g/L or more; clinically overt bleeding requiring transfusion of 2 or more units of whole blood or erythrocytes; intracerebral bleeding; and bleeding involving a critical anatomic site.	**_Age:_** _(Greater 75):_ HR=1.26(95%CI;1.03,1.52)*** **_Comorbidities:_** Hepatic Disease: HR=4.88(95%CI;1.55,15.39)*** **_Other Med Use:_** Aspirin Use: HR=2.41(95%CI;1.69,3.43)*** Statins Use: HR=0.60(95%CI;0.41,0.87)*** **_Warfarin Duration:_** * Cumulative incidence of major bleeding, % (95% CI)* 3 Months: 0.8 (0.5-1.0) 12 Months: 2.6 (2.1-3.2) 24 Months: 4.7 (3.8-5.5)
Douketis 2007[67] Canada Public	Nested case-control study using administrative databases A patients were age 66+ with atrial fibrillation who were prescribed warfarin between April 1, 1994, and December 31, 2001 Follow-up average of 2 years	N(cases): 16,618 (1518) Mean age: 77 (SD=7) 46% Male	Cases were admitted to a hospital with a diagnosis of upper gastrointestinal or intracranial hemorrhage.	**_Other Med Use:_** _Long-term Warfarin Users (>6 months)_ Statins Use: OR=0.82(95%CI;0.67,1.00)*** _Recent Warfarin Users (<6 months)_ Statins Use: OR=1.02(95%CI;0.78,1.34)***

Safe and Effective Anticoagulation in the Outpatient Setting

Study	Design/Population	Sample	Outcome Definition	Results
Fang 2006[64] United States ATRIA Study Public	Cohort study using Administrative Datasets Patients with nonvalvular atrial fibrillation Follow-up 2.4 years (IQR=1.8-2.8)	15,300 person years (170 cases) Mean age: 71 (SD=15) 53% Male	Intracranial hemorrhages unless they were associated with major head trauma (e.g., neurosurgical procedure, motor vehicle accident, and skull fracture). Major extracranial hemorrhages defined as fatal, requiring transfusion of two or more units of packed blood cells, or hemorrhage into a critical anatomic site.	**_New vs. Prior Warfarin_** _Intracranial hemorrhages_ 1st Month: 0.92% /PYr Afterward: 0.46% /PYr RR: 2.0 (95% CI ; 0.6–6.7)* _Major Extracranial hemorrhages_ 1st Month: 1.2% /PYr Afterward: 0.61% /PYr RR: 2.0 (95% CI ; 0.7–5.8)* **_Age_** _Intracranial hemorrhages_ ≥80 v. <80: RR=1.8 (95%CI;1.1–3.1)*** _Major Extracranial hemorrhages_ Per 10 years: RR=1.3 (95%CI;1.1–1.7)***
Fang 2005[59] United States ATRIA Study Public	Cohort study using Administrative Datasets Patients with nonvalvular atrial fibrillation Follow-up 2.4 years (IQR=1.8-2.8)	~15,000 person years (167 cases) Mean age: 71 (SD=15) 53% Male	Intracranial hemorrhages unless they were associated with major head trauma (e.g., neurosurgical procedure, motor vehicle accident, and skull fracture). Major extracranial hemorrhages defined as fatal, requiring transfusion of two or more units of packed blood cells, or hemorrhage into a critical anatomic site.	**_Gender:_** _All major hemorrhages_ Men 1.1% vs. Women 1.0%* Men: RR=1.25 (95% CI;0.91–1.67)*** _Intracranial hemorrhages_ Men 0.55% vs. Women 0.36%* Men: RR=2.0 (95% CI;1.11–3.33)***
Fihn 1996[49] United States - VA National Consortium of Anticoagulation Clinics Government + industry	Combined retrospective and prospective cohort studies Patients attending a combination of VA and university-affiliated clinics anticoagulation clinic between 1980 and 1993 Follow-up: Retrospective study data from 1980 to 1990; prospective study data collected between 1990 and 1993.	N (cases): 2376(259) Mean age: 58.3 73.4% Male	Overt gastrointestinal bleeding; occult gastrointestinal bleeding if endoscopic or radiographic studies were done; gross hematuria prompting cytoscopy or intravenous urography or lasted more than 2 days; hemoptysis.	**_Age group*_** _Serious Bleeding_ RR(95%CI)* <50 yrs: 9.3%/PYr ref 50-59 yrs: 7.1%/PYr 1.2 (0.9-1.6) 60-69 yrs: 6.6%/PYr 1.3 (1.0-1.7) 70-79 yrs: 5.1%/PYr 1.3 (1.0-1.7) 80-89 yrs: 4.4%/PYr 0.9 (0.5-1.5) _Life-threatening or fatal_ RR(95%CI)* <50 yrs: 0.8%/PYr ref 50-59 yrs: 1.3%/PYr 1.3 (0.4-4.1) 60-69 yrs: 1.1%/PYr 1.5 (0.5-4.0) 70-79 yrs: 0.7%/PYr 0.9 (0.3-3.1) 80-89 yrs: 3.4%/PYr 4.5 (1.3-15.6)
Flaker 2006[63] Multinational SPORTIF III & V Trials Industry	Randomized multicenter study (combined open-label and double-blinded studies) High-risk patients with nonvalvular AF Follow-up: 1.4 years (16.5 months) average treatment exposure	N (cases): 3653(125) Mean age: ~71 70% Male	Fatal; involved a critical anatomical site; or overt and associated with a decrease in hemoglobin level of 20 g/L or transfusion of at least 2 U of blood.	**_Warfarin vs Warfarin +aspirin_** (p=.01)* Warfarin (n/N): 2.3% (100/3172) Warfarin + aspirin (n/N): 3.9% (25/481)

Safe and Effective Anticoagulation in the Outpatient Setting

Gage 2006[80] United States NRAF Study Public	Cohort study using medical records from the National registry of Atrial Fibrillation data set. Medicare patients with confirmed atrial fibrillation Follow-up to a maximum of 1000 days after baseline hospitalization	N (cases): 1604(67) Mean age: ~80 ~43% Male	Major bleeding defined using ICD-9-CM codes	*Risk Index (HEMORR₂HAGES)* Bleeds per 100 patient-years (95%CI) Score: 0: 1.9 (0.6-4.4) 1: 2.5 (1.3-4.3) 2: 5.3 (3.4-8.1) 3: 8.4 (4.9-13.6) 4: 10.4 (5.1-18.9) ≥5: 12.3 (5.8-23.1) *Risk Index (OBRI):* Low: 1.1 (0.3-4.3) Moderate: 4.9 (3.6-6.5) High: 8.8 (5.6-14.0) *Risk Index (Kuijer 1999):* Low: 2.9 (1.3-6.5) Moderate: 5.2 (4.0-6.7) High: 7.5 (2.8-19.9) *Risk Index (Kearon 2003):* Score: 0: 2.5 (1.1-6.1) 1: 2.5 (1.4-4.3) 2: 6.5 (4.5-9.4) 3: 9.3 (5.7-15.3) ≥4: 15.3 (6.4-36.8)
Gasse 2005[60] UK Government + industry	Longitudinal cohort study plus a nested case-control analysis Patients (from the UK General Practice research Database) who had a first ever warfarin prescription for AF during the study period and continued treatment for more than 90 days Follow-up was approximately 1 year (3740.8 patient-years of warfarin exposure)	N (cases): 4152(46) Age range: ~70 58% Male	Idiopathic bleeds that resulted in hospitalization within 30 days or death within 7 days following bleeding event	*Warfarin +concomitant drug* [incidence rate = cases/100 PYAR]* Total: 1.2 Warfarin alone: 0.9 Concomitant (all): 1.8 Allopurinol: 3.4 Amiodarone: 1.2 Aspirin: 2.4 Levothyroxine: 0.9 Metronidazole: 38.5 Miconazole: 41.7 Omeprazole: 3.2 Paracetamol: 3.8 Paracetamol + Dextropropoxyphene: 4.1
Gomberg-Maitland 2006[65] Multinational SPORTIF III & V Trials Industry	Randomized multicenter study (combined open-label and double-blinded studies) High-risk patients with nonvalvular AF Followed up to 24 months	N (cases): 3624 (NA) Mean age: ~71 69.7% Male	Major bleeding	*Warfarin arm** Women vs men: -0.35%/yr difference (P=0.491) Men: 91 events, 2.57%/yr Women ≥ 75: 2.60%/yr Women < 75: 1.83%/yr

Safe and Effective Anticoagulation in the Outpatient Setting

Hart 1999[53] Meta-analysis	Meta-analysis of 6 randomized trials of warfarin vs aspirin + warfarin. All published prior to 1998 none of which were largest alone to be included Patients with prosthetic cardiac valves (4 trials), men with coronary risk factors (1 trial), patients with AF (1 trial) Follow-up:	N (cases): 3874(31) Mean age: NA NA % Male	Intracranial hemorrhage	***Warfarin vs Warfarin +aspirin*** (p=.08)* *Warfarin* (n/N): 0.46% (9/1947) *Warfarin + aspirin* (n/N): 1.14% (22/1927)
Healey 2008[69] [ACTIVE-W] Multinational Industry	Prospective randomized study (warfarin arm of RCT) Patients with AF and at least 1 additional risk factor for stroke Followed up to 24 months (median 1.3 years)	N (cases): 3371 (93) Mean age: 70.2 (SD=9.5) 66% Male	Bleeding associated with: death; drop in hemoglobin of at least 2 g/dL; significant hypotension with the need for inotropic agents bleeding requiring surgical intervention (other than vascular site repair); symptomatic intracranial hemorrhage; intraocular hemorrhage causing loss of vison; or the requirement for a transfusion of at least 2 U of blood.	***Risk Index*** (CHADS2 score)* *0:* 0.00/100 pt-yrs *1:* 1.48/100 pt-yrs *2:* 2.89/100 pt-yrs *3:* 2.58/100 pt-yrs *4:* 2.92/100 pt-yrs *5:* 0.90/100 pt-yrs *6:* 6.85/100 pt-yrs *CHADS2=1:* 1.36%/yr *CHADS2>1:* 2.75%/yr ***OAC-naïve**** *CHADS2=1:* 1.81%/yr *CHADS2>1:* 3.76%/yr ***OAC-experienced**** *CHADS2=1:* 1.33%/yr *CHADS2>1:* 2.47%/yr
Higashi 2002[54] United States UWMC Clinics Government + industry	Retrospective cohort study Patients attending Univ of Washington Med Ctr anticoagulation clinics Follow-up: 2.2 years (mean)	N (cases): 185(28) Mean age: 59.9 (SD=15.7) 63.8% Male	Serious bleeding: overt gastrointestinal bleeding; occult gastrointestinal bleeding if endoscopic or radiographic studies were performed; gross hematuria that prompted cystoscopy or intravenous urography or lasted more than 2 days; hemoptysis; blood transfusions of 2 units or more.	***CYP2C9 Genotype**** *Variant:* 10.92% /PYr *Wild-type:* 4.89% /PYr
Johnson 2008[70] United States Public	Retrospective longitudinal cohort study: warfarin vs warfarin + antiplatelet combination therapy Patients attending Kaiser Permanente Colorado anticoagulation clinics Follow-up: 4.6 yr (SD=4.0)	N (cases): 4183(55) Mean age: 70.7(SD=12.5 53.3% Male	Major hemorrhage: required the transfusion of two or more units of RBCs; caused a decrease in hemoglobin concentration of ≥ 2 g/dL; or involved any intracranial, intraarticular, intraocular, or retroperitoneal sites	***Warfarin vs Warfarin + antiplatelet*** (p=.003)* *Warfarin* (n/N): 0.9% (23/2560) *Warfarin + antiplatelet* (n/N): 2.0% (32/1623)

Safe and Effective Anticoagulation in the Outpatient Setting

Study	Description	N (cases)	Outcome	Results
Le Tourneau 2009[81] United States Public	Population-based retrospective cohort study with chart review Patients in Olmsted County, MN who had mechanical mitral value replacement Follow-up: 8.2 yr (SD=6.1)	N (cases): 112(27) Mean age: 57 (SD=16) 40% Male	Bleeding causing death, hospitalization, permanent injury or transfusion	*Cancer HR 4.01 (95%CI; 1.89-8.52)*** *INR SD (Variability)* HR 2.48 (95%CI; 1.11-5.55)**
Limdi 2008[71] United States POAT Study Public	Prospective cohort study: influence of genotypes on risk for hemorrhagic complications Patients participating in the Pharmacogenetic Optimization of Anticoagulation Therapy (POAT) cohort study Follow-up: 14.9 mo (SD=10.7)	N (cases): 446(44) Mean age: 60.6 (SD=15.6) 51.3% Male 50.9% African American	Major hemorrhage	*Incidence rate by genotype** *CYP2C9* *Total:* 7.93/100 PYr *Wild type:* 5.67/100 PYr *Variant:* 15.74/100 PYr *VKORC1 1173C/T* *Total:* 8.0/100 PYr *"CC":* 7.4/100 PYr *Any "T":* 8.9/100 PYr
Limdi 2009[75] United States POAT Study Public	Secondary analysis of a prospective cohort study: influence of kidney function on risk for hemorrhagic complications Patients participating in the Pharmacogenetic Optimization of Anticoagulation Therapy (POAT) cohort study Follow-up: 16.2 mo (mean)	N (cases): 565(64) Mean age: 61 (SD=16) 51.1% Male 47.6% African American	Major hemorrhage	*Incidence rate by GFR** *Overall:* 8.4/100 PYr *GFR≥60:* 6.2/100 PYr *GFR=30-59:* 8.3/100 PYr *GFR<30:* 30.5/100 PYr
Lind 2009[77] Sweden Public	Prospective cohort study Patients with at least a 3 month duration treatment plan were recruited from several warfarin clinics Follow-up: 4.2 years	N(cases): 719(73) Mean age: 70 (SD=11) 63% Male	Fatal bleeding and/or symptomatic bleeding in a critical area or organ and/or bleeding causing a fall in hemoglobin level of 2 g/dL or more	*Unadjusted* *Gender:** Men: RR=0.8 (95% CI;0.5–1.2) *hsCRP:** Per 1 SD: 1.0 (95% CI;0.8–1.3) *MV Adjusted* **Age***** Per 10 years: RR=1.4 (95%CI;1.1–1.7) *Thrombomodulin:**** Per 1 SD: 1.4 (95% CI;1.2–1.7)

Safe and Effective Anticoagulation in the Outpatient Setting

Study	Design / Population	Outcome Definition	N(cases) / Demographics	Results
Lindh 2008[72] Sweden WARG (Warfarin Genetics) study Public and Industry	Prospective cohort with nested case-control for association of INR and severe bleeding risk No restriction on indication for warfarin treatment Starting warfarin treatment or on anticoagulant for < 2 wks Study period: 12/2001 – 8/2005 1276 patient-years follow-up	WHO criteria: lethal, life-threatening, permanently disabling, or leading to hospital admission (ED admissions excluded) or prolongation of hospital stay	N(cases): 1523(33 in 29 patients) Median (interquartile range) age: 66 (57; 74) 63% Male	*First 165 days of treatment vs. beyond 165* RR 1.1 (95%CI; 0.5-2.3) *First treatment month vs. beyond 1 month* RR 2.4 (95%CI; 1.0-6.0) **Age** HR 1.02 (95%CI; 0.98-1.06)*** **Male sex** HR 2.8 (95%CI; 1.1-7.3)*** *Target INR* HR 1.3 (95%CI; 0.03-50)*** *Aver. Warfarin Dose (mg/d)* HR 0.97 (95%CI; 0.79-1.2)*** *Time Outside Ther. INR interval* HR 1.2 (95%CI; 0.95-1.5)*** *Interacting drugs at start of tx (yes/no)* HR 2.3 (95%CI; 1.1-4.9)*** *INR at time of event (28cases:56 controls)* OR 1.9 (95%CI; 1.1-3.4)
McMahan 1998[52] United States, Veteran's Affairs Medical Center Funding NR	Retrospective cohort No restriction on indication for warfarin therapy Most recent course of treatment (if multiple courses) Followed from start of treatment at VAMC between 3/31/89 and 3/31/94 to end of treatment or 7/1/94; mean duration of follow-up 14.0 mos (range: 1 day to 60 mos)	Landefeld's bleeding severity index – major hemorrhage defined based on patient survival, amount of blood lost, and physical consequences of the hemorrhage	N(cases): 565(40) Mean Age 65.1 (SD=10.9) 98.5% Male	*GI bleeding* RR 2.1 (95%CI; 0.93-4.9)*** *Comorbid Condition* RR 1.6 (95%CI; 0.86-3.1)*** *Stroke* RR 1.2 (95%CI; 0.50-2.9)*** **Age ≥65 yrs** RR 1.0 (95%CI; 0.53-1.9)*** *Atrial Fibrillation* RR 1.0 (95%CI; 0.47-2.1)*** *Alcohol abuse* RR 2.7 (95%CI; 1.4-5.4)*** *Chronic renal insufficiency* RR 2.6 (95%CI; 1.3-5.2)*** *Previous GI bleed* RR 2.4 (95%CI;1.1-6.0)*** *NOTE: other factor not significant in univariate analyses include: gender(p=.63), NSAID (p=.78), aspirin (p=.56), diabetes (p=.27)*
Meckley 2008[73] United States UWMC Clinics Government + industry	Retrospective cohort of patients attending Univ of Washington Med Ctr anticoagulation clinics No restriction on indication for warfarin therapy; had known *CYP2C9* and *VKORC1* genotype status Attended anticoagulation clinic between 4/3/90 and 4/21/01 with confirmed initial warfarin exposure date and at least 2 clinic visits Excluded Asian or African race	Serious and life-threatening bleeds according to Fihn, 1993 definition	N(cases): 172(31) Mean age: 59.8 64.5% Male	**Genetics*** *CYP2C9 (Variant vs Wild-type)* HR 3.18 (95%CI; 1.30-7.78) *VKORC1 (vs. AB)* *AA:* HR 1.21 (95%CI; 0.38-3.82) *BB:* HR 0.83 (95%CI; 0.33-2.09)

Safe and Effective Anticoagulation in the Outpatient Setting

Study	Design / Setting	Outcome	N(cases) / Demographics	Results
Metlay 2008[74] United States Public	Prospective cohort No restriction on indication for warfarin therapy New and continuing users of warfarin; over age 65 Recruited between 5/1/02 and 5/31/03; 24 month follow-up	Any hospitalization due to warfarin-related bleeding (meeting specified criteria and reviewed by independent reviewers)	N(cases): 2370 (111) Mean age: ~78 (all over 65) 23% Male	**_Duration of Warfarin Use*_** _New users of warfarin:_ 4.5/100 PY (95% CI; 2.9-6.8) _Chronic users of warfarin:_ 4.7/100PY (95%CI; 3.7-5.8) _First month of follow-up vs. all other months:*_ RR 0.9 (95%CI; 0.4-1.8) **_Age_** No association*** **_Meds_** _NSAID/ASA (vs. neither)***_ RR 1.4 (95%CI; 0.9-2.1) _Number of Current medications (vs. 1-3 meds)***_ 4-8 Meds: RR 1.5 (95%CI; 0.8-3.0) ≥9 Meds: RR 2.2 (95%CI; 1.0-4.6) **_Primary Indication***_ _Valve condition requiring warfarin (vs. other indications):_ RR 3.02 (95%CI; 1.91-4.78) _Anticoagulation clinic (vs. non-specialized clinic):_ RR 1.63 (95%CI 0.84-3.14)
Poli 2009b[78] Italy Funding NR	Prospective cohort Atrial fibrillation Referred to anticoagulation clinic between 6/98 and 12/07 2,365 pt/years follow-up; median time of follow-up 3.1 years (range: 3 mos-9.5 yrs)	Fatal, intracranial, ocular causing blindness, articular, or retroperitoneal; surgery or transfusion of >2 blood units required; hemoglobin reduced 2 g/dl or more	N(cases): 662 (32 with 17 cerebral) Median age: 75 yrs (range: 49-94) 64% Male	**_Risk Index (AFI):*_** _Low:_ 0 _Moderate:_ 1.3/100 PY _High:_ 1.4/100 PY **_Risk Index (ACCP):*_** _Low:_ 0 _Moderate:_ 0 _High_ 1.4/100 PY **_Risk Index (CHADS2):*_** _Low:_ 0 _Moderate:_ 1.0/100 PY _High:_ 1.9/100 PY **_Risk Index (NICE):*_** _Low:_ 0 _Moderate:_ 1.0/100 PY _High:_ 1.5/100 PY
Poli 2009a[76] Italy Funding NR	Prospective cohort Atrial fibrillation Referred to anticoagulation clinic between 6/98 and 12/07 2,567 pt/years follow-up; mean time of follow-up 2.7 years (range: 0.1 -13 yrs)	Fatal, intracranial, ocular causing blindness, articular, or retroperitoneal; surgery or transfusion of >2 blood units required; hemoglobin reduced 2 g/dl or more	N(cases): 783 (37 with 20 cerebral) Median age: 75 yrs (range: 37-94) 65% Male	**_Age:*_** _Major bleeding_ ≥80 v. <80: RR=1.9 (95%CI;1.2-2.8) _Cerebral bleeding_ ≥80 v. <80: RR=2.1 (95%CI;0.8-5.5)

Schauer 2005[61] United States Public	Retrospective cohort Nonvalvular atrial fibrillation Ohio Medicaid patients; 1/1/97 to 5/31/02 Mean follow-up 740 days	N(cases): 9,345 (1022) Mean age: 72 (SD=13.8) 32% Male	Intracranial hemorrhage, and gastrointestinal bleeding requiring hospitalization	
			Intracranial Hemorrhage:	HR (95% CI)
			Substance abuse	2.4 (1.4, 4.0)***
			Psychiatric illness	1.5 (1.0, 2.1) ***
			Social risk factors	0.9 (0.7, 1.3) *
			Hypertension	1.4 (0.9, 2.2) *
			CHF	0.9 (0.6, 1.2) *
			Diabetes mellitus	0.9 (0.7, 1.3) *
			Liver disease	0.9 (0.4, 2.0) *
			Renal disease	1.3 (0.9, 1.9) *
			DVT	0.9 (0.6, 1.5) *
			Age (per decade)	1.0 (0.9, 1.2) *
			Sex, male	1.1 (0.8, 1.5) *
			Race, white	0.8 (0.6, 1.2) *
			GI Bleeding:	HR (95% CI)
			Substance abuse	1.4 (1.1, 1.9)***
			Psychiatric illness	1.2 (1.0, 1.4) ***
			Social risk factors	1.3 (1.1, 1.5) ***
			Hypertension	1.1 (1.0, 1.3) *
			CHF	1.3 (1.1, 1.6) *
			Diabetes	1.0 (0.9, 1.2) *
			Liver disease	1.3 (1.0, 1.7) ***
			Renal disease	1.6 (1.4, 1.9) ***
			DVT	1.2 (1.0, 1.5) ***
			Age (per decade)	1.0 (1.0, 1.1) *
			Sex, male	1.1 (0.9, 1.2) *
			Race, white	0.9 (0.7, 1.0) *

Safe and Effective Anticoagulation in the Outpatient Setting

Schelleman 2010[79] United States Non-profit	Case-control study nested within the Medicaid programs Evaluating new antihyperlipidemic prescriptions in patients on warfarin for at least 90 days California, Florida, New York, Ohio, and Pennsylvania Medicaid patients from 1999 to 2003 Average follow-up appears to be nearly 1 year	Total N=353,489 Cases=12,193 Mean age: ~69 33% Male	ICD-9 code indicating hospitalization for gastrointestinal bleeding.	**GI Bleeding**

	OR (95% CI)***
New Prescription	
Fenofibrate	No data
Gemfibrozil	1.96 (1.19-3.24)
Fluvastatin	1.45 (0.68-3.09)
Simvastatin	1.33 (1.00-1.78)
Atorvastatin	1.29 (1.04-1.61)
Pravastatin	0.66 (0.38-1.14)
3rd to 4th Prescription	OR (95% CI)***
Fenofibrate	1.31 (0.62-2.79)
Gemfibrozil	1.23 (0.61-2.48)
Fluvastatin	No data
Simvastatin	1.10 (0.79-1.53)
Atorvastatin	0.62 (0.46-0.85)
Pravastatin	0.54 (0.29-1.01)
	OR (95% CI)*
Male sex	0.95 (0.92-0.99)
Age, (ref=<50)	
50-59	1.43 (1.32-1.56)
60-69	1.81 (1.68-1.96)
70-79	2.14 (1.99-2.30)
80+	2.34 (2.18-2.51)
Prior GI bleed	3.12 (3.00-3.24)
Diabetes	1.62 (1.56-1.68)
Liver disease	1.79 (1.72-1.87)
CKD	2.57 (2.47-2.68)

Study	Design / Population	N (cases)	Outcome	Results
Shireman 2006[66] United States Non-profit	Retrospective Cohort Atrial fibrillation All patients ≥ 65 years old; discharged from hospital receiving warfarin therapy between 4/98 and 3/99 and between 7/00 and 6/01	Total N=26,345 (~415) Development cohort n=19,875 (~318) Validation cohort n=6,470(~97) Mean age: 88% 70 years or older 47% Male	Hospitalized for major acute bleeding event (GI hemorrhage, intracranial hemorrhage) (NOTE: only included events within 90 days of discharge from index AF admission and only the first event for a subject)	**<u>Results from Development Cohort</u>** *Age ≥ 70 yrs:* HR 1.63 (95%CI: 1.08-2.48) *Male gender:* HR 0.73 (95%CI: 0.58-0.92) *Remote bleeding event:* HR 1.79 (95%CI; 1.36-2.37) *Recent bleeding event:* HR 1.85 (95%CI; 1.41-2.44) *Alcohol or drug abuse:* HR 2.03 (95%CI; 1.07-3.83) *Diabetes:* HR 1.31 (95%CI; 1.04-1.66) *Anemia:* HR 2.36 (95%CI; 1.76-3.17) *Antiplatelet drug:* HR 1.38 (95%CI 1.07-1.78) **<u>Results from Validation Cohort</u>** <u>*Risk Index (Shireman 2006):* (p<0.0001)</u> *Low: 0.9% (cases=35)* *Moderate: 2.0% (cases=48)* *High: 5.4% (cases=12)* <u>*Risk Index (Kuijer 1999): (p=0.74)*</u> *Moderate: 1.5%* *High: 1.8%* <u>*Risk Index (OBRI): (p<0.0001)*</u> *Moderate: 1.0%* *High: 2.5%*
Smith 2002[55] United States Public	Case-control Cases: history of stroke, taking warfarin, and hospitalized for warfarin-related ICH; age ≥ 60 Controls: history of stroke, taking warfarin, age ≥ 60 80% of each group treated with warfarin as a result of previous stroke or TIA	N(cases): 82(26) Mean age: 75 53 % Male	Intracranial hemorrhage	**<u>Comorbidity</u>** <u>*Leukoaraiosis:*</u> OR 12.9 (95%CI;2.8-59.8); adjusted OR 8.4 (95%CI; 1.4-51.5) <u>*Severe (grade 3 or 4) leukoaraiosis:*</u> OR 24.9 (95%CI;4.5-137.4) vs. absence of leukoaraiosis
Stroke Prevention in Atrial Fibrillation (SPAF) Investigators 1996[48] United States SPAF II study Public	Warfarin arm of RCT comparing warfarin and aspirin Non-valvular atrial fibrillation Candidates for warfarin anticoagulation Mean follow-up 2.6 years	N(cases): 555(34) Mean age: 70 for all patients 69% Male	Bleeding involving the central nervous system; requiring hospitalization, blood transfusion, and/or surgical intervention; or resulted in permanent functional impairment to any degree	<u>*Univariate Risk of Bleeding During Warfarin Treatment:*</u>* **Age > 75 yr:** RR 2.6 (p=0.009) **Male gender:** RR 0.9 **Comorbidities** *Thromboembolism:* RR 1.9 *CHF:* RR 2.0 (p=0.05) *Diabetes:* RR 1.9 (p=0.09) *GI bleeding:* RR 1.6 *Hypertension:* RR 1.1 **Other Meds** *NSAIDs:* RR 1.3 *Other prescriptions:* RR 1.2/drug (p=0.003) **Other** *Tobacco Use:* RR 1.9 (p=0.1) *Alcohol:* RR 1.0

			INR Time in Range and Variability:**
Van Leeuwen 2008[82] The Netherlands LAVA study Funding NR	Case-control study nested within a cohort of patients with prosthetic heart valves treated in four anticoagulation clinics between 1985-1993 Cases had a hemorrhagic event during follow-up. Controls were matched 2 per case on age and sex.	N(cases): 460(154)	Hemorrhagic events included: intracranial and spinal hemorrhage; or major extracranial hemorrhage leading to death or hospitalization (except hemorrhage that led to hospital admission for diagnostic procedures only).	In range & stable = Reference In range & unstable: OR 1.0 (0.5-2.0) Outrange & stable: OR 1.6 (0.9-3.1) Outrange & unstable: OR 2.7 (1.4-4.9)
White 1996[50] United States - VA National Consortium of Anticoagulation Clinics Government + industry	Retrospective review of patients followed in clinics during 4/89 Prospective follow-up of all patients with life-threatening bleeding during retrospective review AND all patients between 6/90 and 4/93 Patients treated with warfarin for at least 6 weeks No restriction on indication for warfarin therapy 3,865 PY of follow-up	N(cases): 1,999 (32) Mean age: 58.79 (SD=14.3) 75.3% Male	Life-threatening: cardiopulmon-ary arrest, surgical or angio-graphic intervention to stop the bleeding, irreversible sequelae (including MI, ICH, blindness, or fibrothroax), or any 2 of the following: transfusion of ≥ 3 U of blood, hypotension, critical anemia, or acute bleeding	Male gender:* 21 of 32 bleeding cases (66%) vs. 75.3% of study population Primary Indication* Mechanical valve: 17/32 (53%) vs. 20% of study population VTE: 5/32 (16%) vs. 23.9% of study population Atrial fibrillation: 6/32 (19%) vs. 16.9% of study population

Risk Factor categories (* = Unadjusted; ** = Adjusted for Age and/or basic demographics like gender; ***=multivariable adjustment for other covariates thought to be related to serious bleeding).
/PYr =per patient year